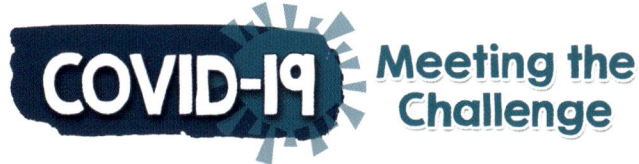

COVID-19 Meeting the Challenge

Making Communities Resilient to Pandemics

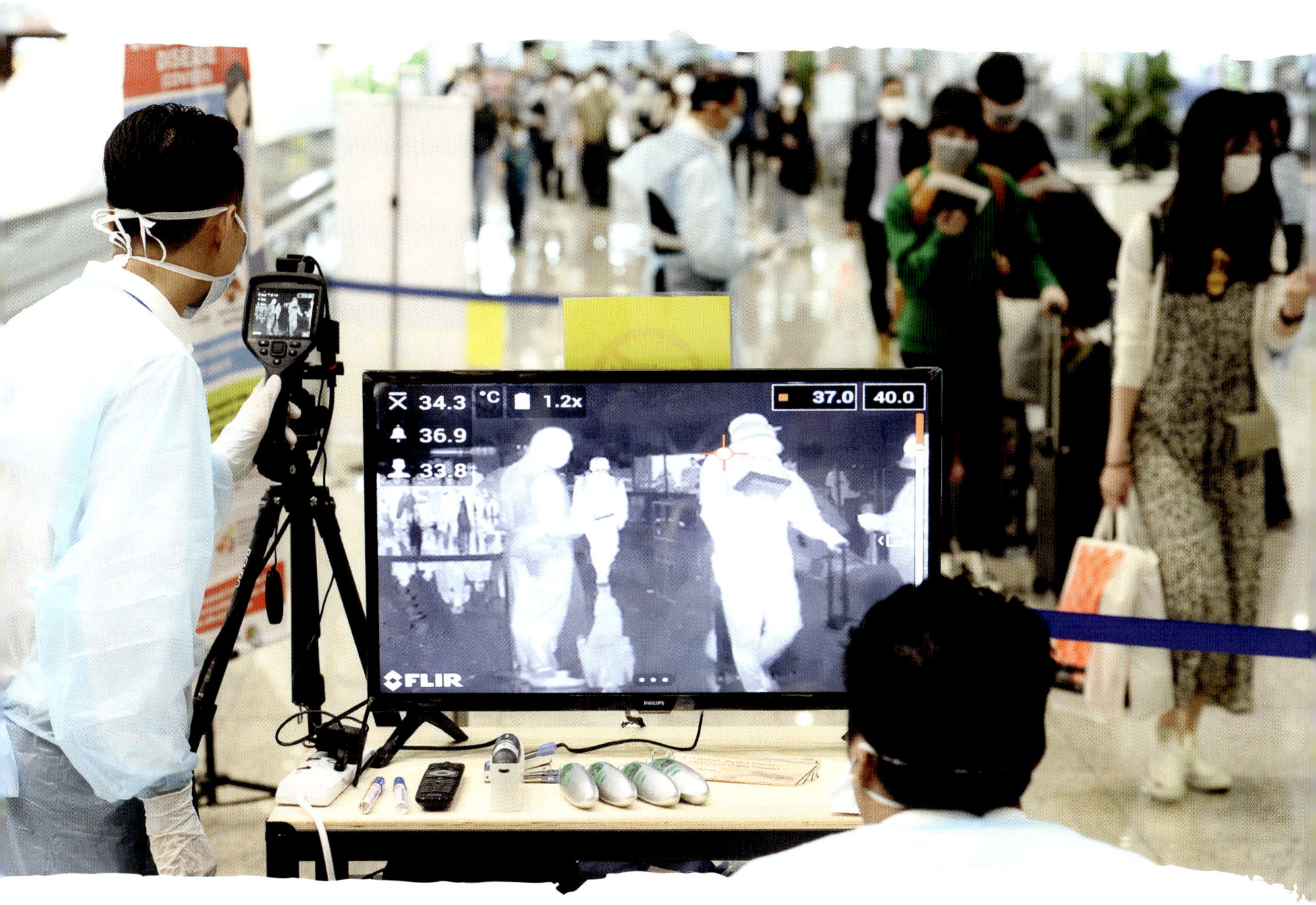

Linda Barghoorn

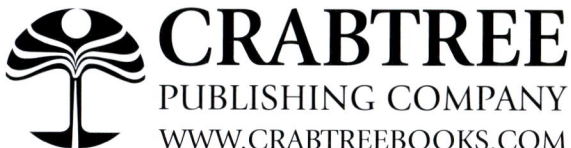

CRABTREE PUBLISHING COMPANY
WWW.CRABTREEBOOKS.COM

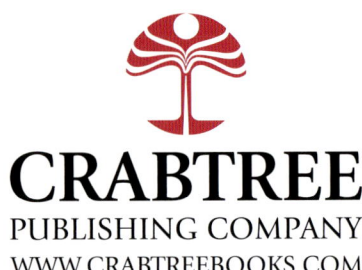

CRABTREE PUBLISHING COMPANY
WWW.CRABTREEBOOKS.COM

Author:
Linda Barghoorn

Series research and development:
Janine Deschenes and Ellen Rodger

Editorial director:
Kathy Middleton

Editors:
Ellen Rodger and Janine Deschenes

Proofreader:
Wendy

Graphic design:
Samara Parent

Image research:
Samara Parent

Print coordinator:
Katherine Berti

Images:
Alamy
  The Protected Art Archive: p. 6-7
  Sueddeutsche Zeitung Photo: p. 10-11
  B Christopher: p. 25 (bottom)
  BJ Warnick: p. 26 (bottom)

Getty Image
  Getty STR: p. 4–5

Shutterstock
  Daria Nipot: front cover (top left)
  lev radin: front cover (top left)
  FiledIMAGE: front cover (bottom)
  NAUFAL ZAQUAN: title page
  YL Stock: p. 3
  Lesia Povkh: p. 12 (top)
  Chirag Nagpal: p. 14 (bottom)
  Marius Dobilas: p. 14-15
  Sumit Saraswat: p. 17
  Wirestock Creators: p. 18 (bottom)
  Ryan DeBerardinis: p. 18-19
  Suzanne C. Grim: p. 20-21
  Sorbis: p. 22 (bottom)
  Vic Hinterlang: p. 22-23
  chrisdorney: p. 24 (middle right)
  MikeDotta: p. 24 (bottom)
  Somphop Krittayaworagul: p. 25 (top)
  photo-lime: p. 26-27
  Wut_Moppie: p. 28
  TK Kurikawa: p. 29 (top)
  Adam Calaitzis: p. 29 (bottom)
  Tommy Larey: p. 33

Adam Yesner: p. 34
Arief Budi Kusuma: p. 37 (top)
hairul_nizam: p. 38 (bottom)
Kristi Blokhin: p. 40
lev radin: p. 41
MikeDotta: p. 42
Nach-Noth: p. 43
Aleksandr Dyskin: p. 45

Wikimedia Commons
  TxllxT TxllxT: p. 9

Image courtesy of SUNY Downstate Health Sciences University: p. 39 (bottom)

All other images by Shutterstock

Library and Archives Canada Cataloguing in Publication

Title: Making communities resilient to pandemics / Linda Barghoorn.
Names: Barghoorn, Linda, author.
Description: Series statement: COVID-19: meeting the challenge | Includes bibliographical references and index.
Identifiers: Canadiana (print) 20210214775 | Canadiana (ebook) 20210214783 | ISBN 9781427156037 (hardcover) | ISBN 9781427156051 (softcover) | ISBN 9781427156075 (HTML) | ISBN 9781427156396 (EPUB)
Subjects: LCSH: COVID-19 Pandemic, 2020—Social aspects—Juvenile literature. | LCSH: Epidemics—Social aspects—History—Juvenile literature. | LCSH: Epidemics—Prevention—Juvenile literature. | LCSH: City and town life—Health aspects—Juvenile literature.
Classification: LCC RA644.C67 B37 2022 | DDC j614.5/92414—dc23

Library of Congress Cataloging-in-Publication Data

Names: Barghoorn, Linda, author.
Title: Making communities resilient to pandemics / Linda Barghoorn.
Description: New York, NY : Crabtree Publishing Company, [2022] | Series: COVID-19: meeting the challenge | Includes bibliographical references and index.
Identifiers: LCCN 2021020729 (print) | LCCN 2021020730 (ebook) | ISBN 9781427156037 (hardcover) | ISBN 9781427156051 (paperback) | ISBN 9781427156075 (ebook) | ISBN 9781427156396 (epub)
Subjects: LCSH: Urban health--Juvenile literature. | City planning--Health aspects--Juvenile literature. | Public health--Juvenile literature. | COVID-19 (Disease)--Juvenile literature.
Classification: LCC RA566.7 .B366 2022 (print) | LCC RA566.7 (ebook) | DDC 362.1/042--dc23
LC record available at https://lccn.loc.gov/2021020729
LC ebook record available at https://lccn.loc.gov/2021020730

Crabtree Publishing Company

www.crabtreebooks.com 1-800-387-7650

Copyright © **2022 CRABTREE PUBLISHING COMPANY**. All rights reserved. No part of this publication may be reproduced, stored in a retrieval system or be transmitted in any form or by any means, electronic, mechanical, photocopying, recording, or otherwise, without the prior written permission of Crabtree Publishing Company. In Canada: We acknowledge the financial support of the Government of Canada through the Canada Book Fund for our publishing activities.

Published in Canada
Crabtree Publishing
616 Welland Ave.
St. Catharines, Ontario
L2M 5V6

Published in the United States
Crabtree Publishing
347 Fifth Ave
Suite 1402-145
New York, NY 10016

Printed in the U.S.A./092021/CG20210616

CONTENTS

Introduction 4

Chapter 1
Throughout History 6

Chapter 2
The COVID-19 Pandemic 14

Chapter 3
The Need for Resilience 20

Chapter 4
Resilience Strategies 26

Chapter 5
Building Resilient Communities 34

Bibliography 44

Timeline 45

Learning More 46

Glossary 46

Index 48

About the Author 48

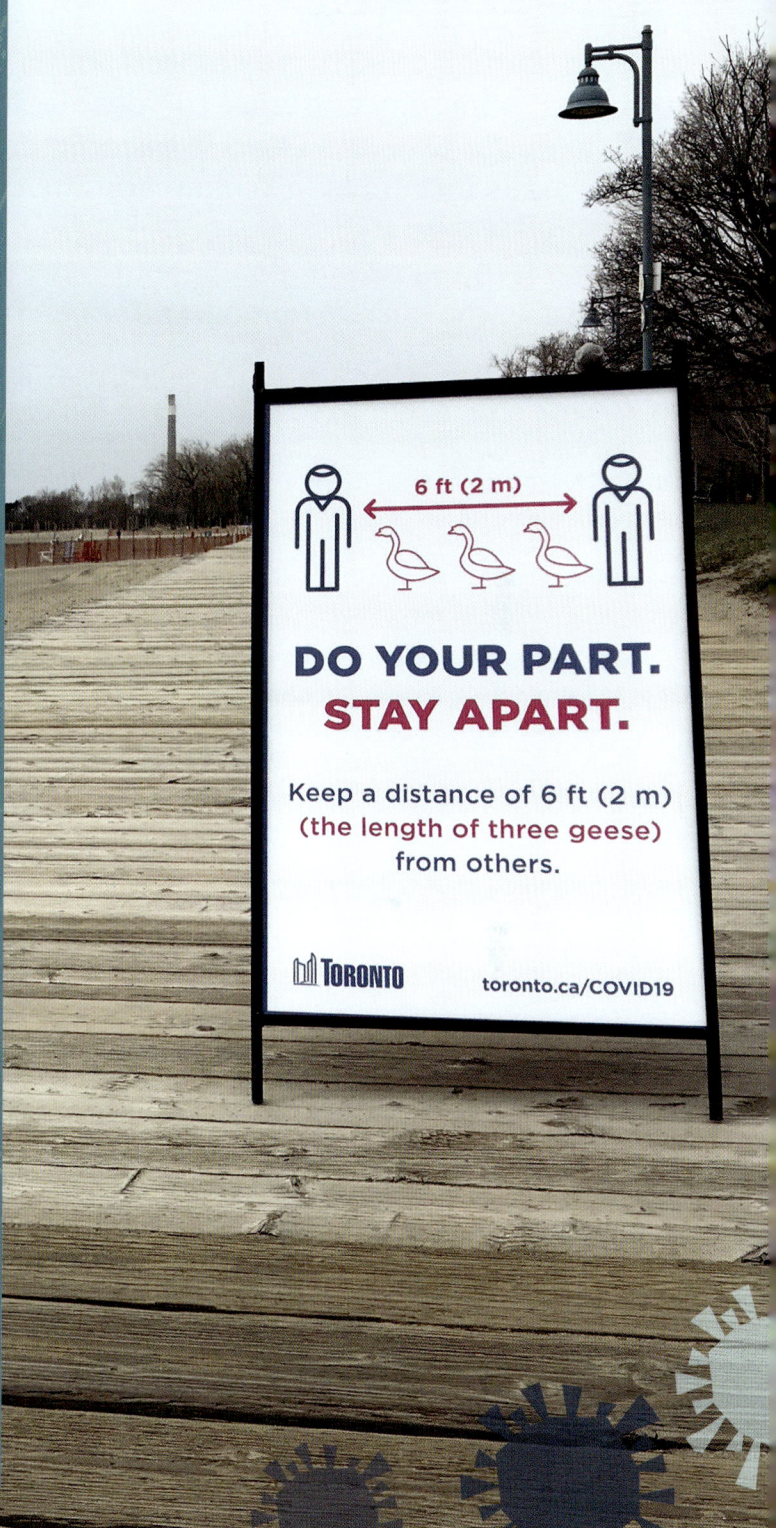

Introduction

In the final weeks of 2019, a mysterious illness began to spread among the citizens of Wuhan, China. Doctors struggled to identify and treat the deadly, flu-like virus. On January 23, 2020, the Chinese government announced an enormous **lockdown** in Wuhan and the cities around it. The goal was to try to control the spread of the disease. More than 60 million people were forced into **quarantine**—the largest number in human history.

The Chinese government was determined to win the fight against the virus. It put extreme measures in place. All personal travel was forbidden. Roads leading into and out of Wuhan were blocked. Flights, trains, and public transit were canceled. Schools, factories, and businesses were closed. Emergency **field hospitals** were built to handle the number of patients overwhelming the hospitals.

Only shops selling food or medicine were allowed to stay open. People were told to stay in their homes, with only one family member allowed to leave for groceries. Security guards stood at checkpoints at building entrances. They restricted anyone from entering or leaving without permission.

Officials led door-to-door health checks on citizens. Anyone showing signs of illness was taken away to a quarantine facility. Drones with loudspeakers monitored citizens' movements, scolding anyone not following the rules. Medical supplies ran short and doctors felt the strain of long hours and difficult conditions. The streets became eerily quiet. Months would pass before people were allowed to emerge and begin rebuilding their lives.

Wuhan's strict lockdown ended in April 2020. The city held a massive pool party to celebrate zero COVID-19 cases on August 17, 2020.

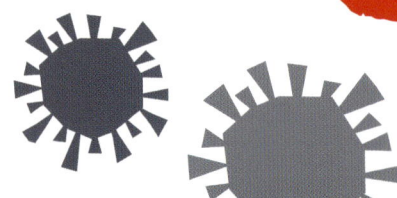

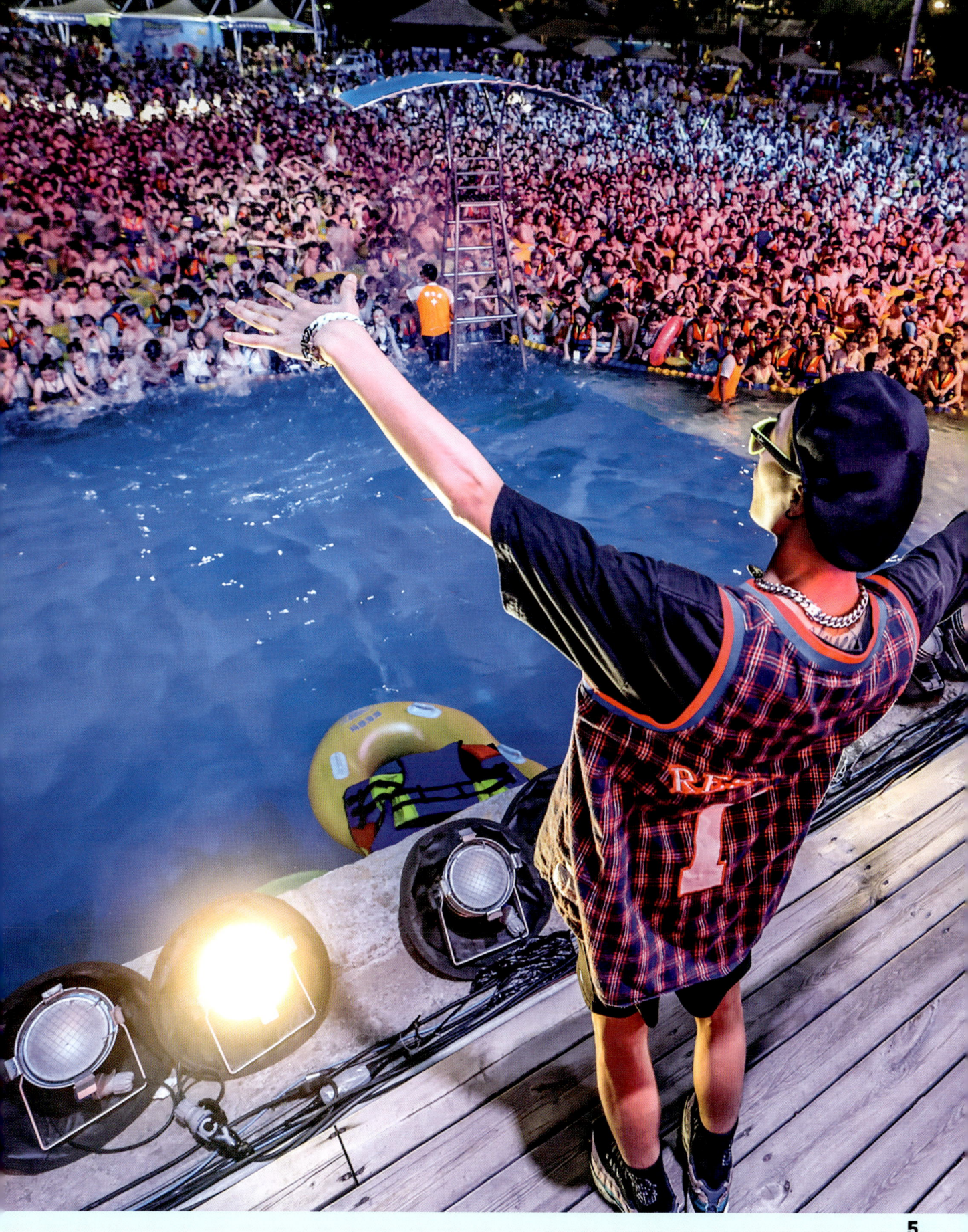

Chapter 1

Throughout History

Viruses and diseases have been among us for thousands of years—killing more people than all the wars throughout history. Pandemics have destroyed **empires**, ruined **economies**, and spread panic.

The Plague of Athens

When an **epidemic** swept through the crowded ancient city of Athens in 430 BCE, almost half the city's population died. Panic spread among the survivors. As they lost faith that their leaders could protect them, they refused to support the government and its rules. Society began to crumble. Although the city managed to survive, its empire was destroyed.

The word quarantine comes from the Italian term "quaranta giorni," meaning 40 days. It referred to the practice, started in the 1300s, of keeping passengers on ships for 40 days before they enter a city. This helped prevent the spread of disease.

The Black Death, or bubonic plague, was a pandemic that swept through Asia, Europe, and Africa in the 1300s. Caused by the bite of an infected flea, the disease killed an estimated 50 million people worldwide.

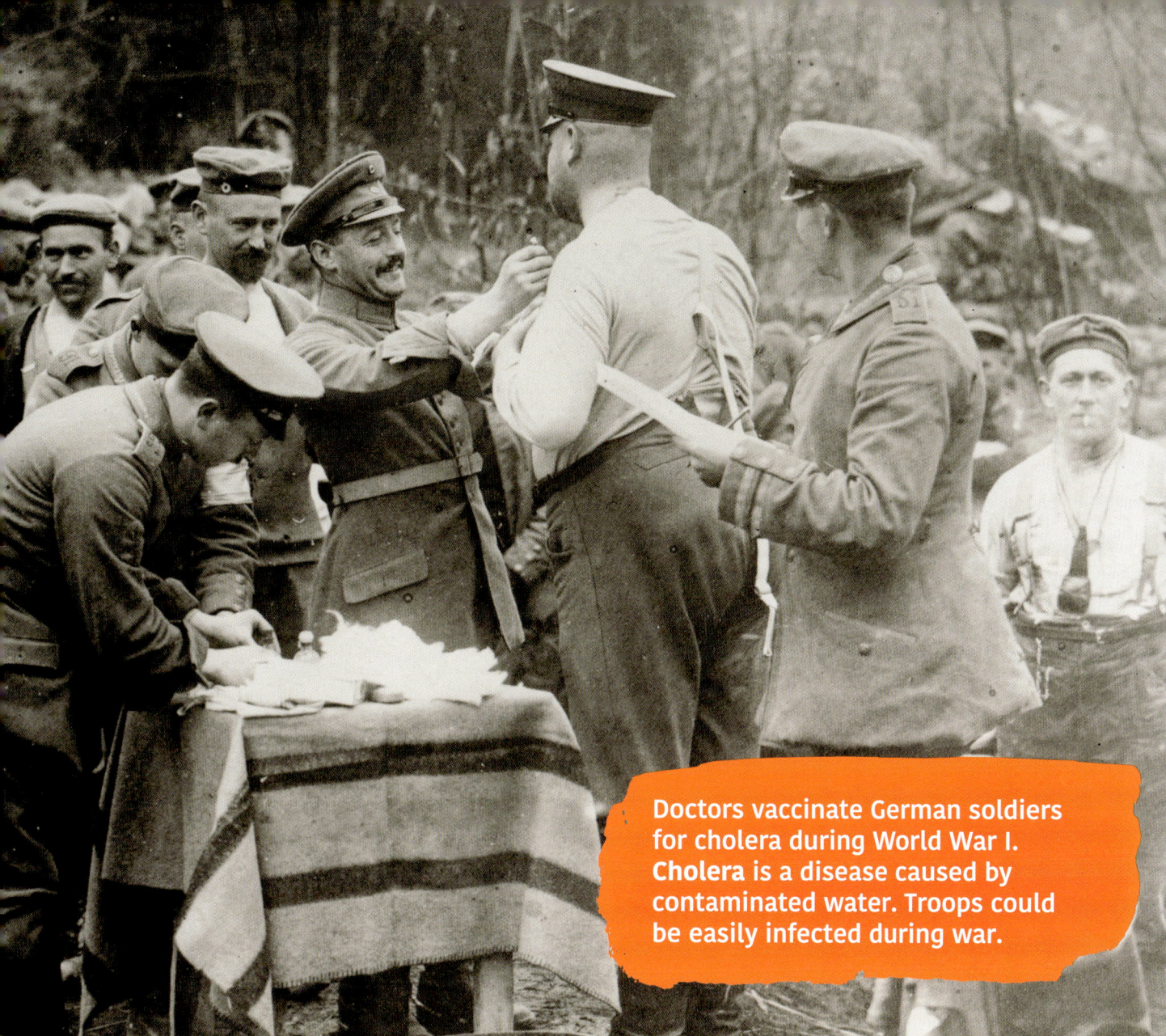

Doctors vaccinate German soldiers for cholera during World War I. **Cholera** is a disease caused by contaminated water. Troops could be easily infected during war.

The Black Death

In 1347, 12 ships arrived in the port city of Messina, on the Mediterranean island of Sicily. Many sailors on board were sick or dead. Authorities ordered the ships to leave, but it was too late. As the mysterious disease spread across Europe, people fled the cities. Thousands more were killed in an effort to rid the cities of evil. It was believed that God had sent the disease to punish evil citizens. In fact, the plague had been carried by flea-infested rats aboard the ships. More than 20 million people died in one of the deadliest pandemics ever.

Cholera Breakout

In the 1800s, the German seaport city of Hamburg was run by a group of families whose fortunes relied on trade. When a **cholera** epidemic broke out in 1892, they refused to admit what was happening. They were more worried about how the disease would hurt business. When the city was finally forced into quarantine, its reputation suffered and trade collapsed. It took years for Hamburg to recover. That recovery only occurred after a safe water supply and regular inspections for cleanliness were guaranteed.

Rural to Urban

For much of history, the world's population was **rural**. People lived and worked on farms. In the 1800s, millions of people moved from the countryside to cities in search of better-paying jobs. Those cities looked very different from the modern cities we live in today. They were often dirty, over-crowded, and filled with diseases. There were no facilities to provide clean water or remove waste and garbage. Housing was in short supply, so poorly built **slums** sprung up to house factory workers and their families.

Early Disease Prevention

Dirty water, untreated sewage, and poor living conditions meant that disease was common and difficult to control. There were no health care systems in place to help people. Millions of people died in epidemics caused by influenza, cholera, smallpox, and other **infectious** diseases.

Clean Water

Eventually, those outbreaks forced city leaders to look at health issues and improve living conditions. Building codes helped fix overcrowding problems. **Sanitation** services provided people with clean water, garbage removal, and systems to remove sewage from homes. Health authorities were created to develop guidelines and programs for **public health**. Modern medicines were invented to treat infections and disease. They have played an important role in defeating diseases that had once devastated cities.

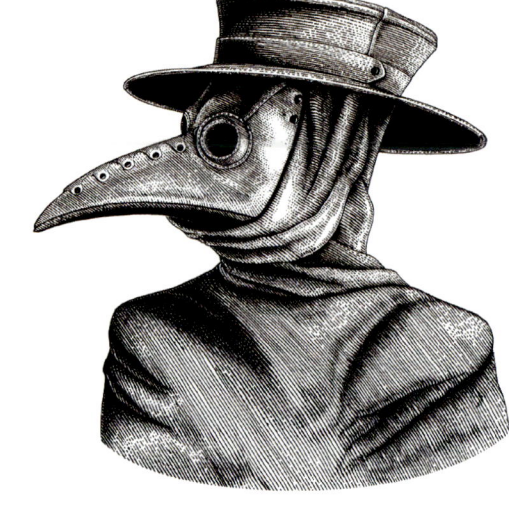

Plague doctors were hired by towns and cities to treat victims of the bubonic plague. They wore special masks with long beaks stuffed with herbs and leaves believed to ward off disease.

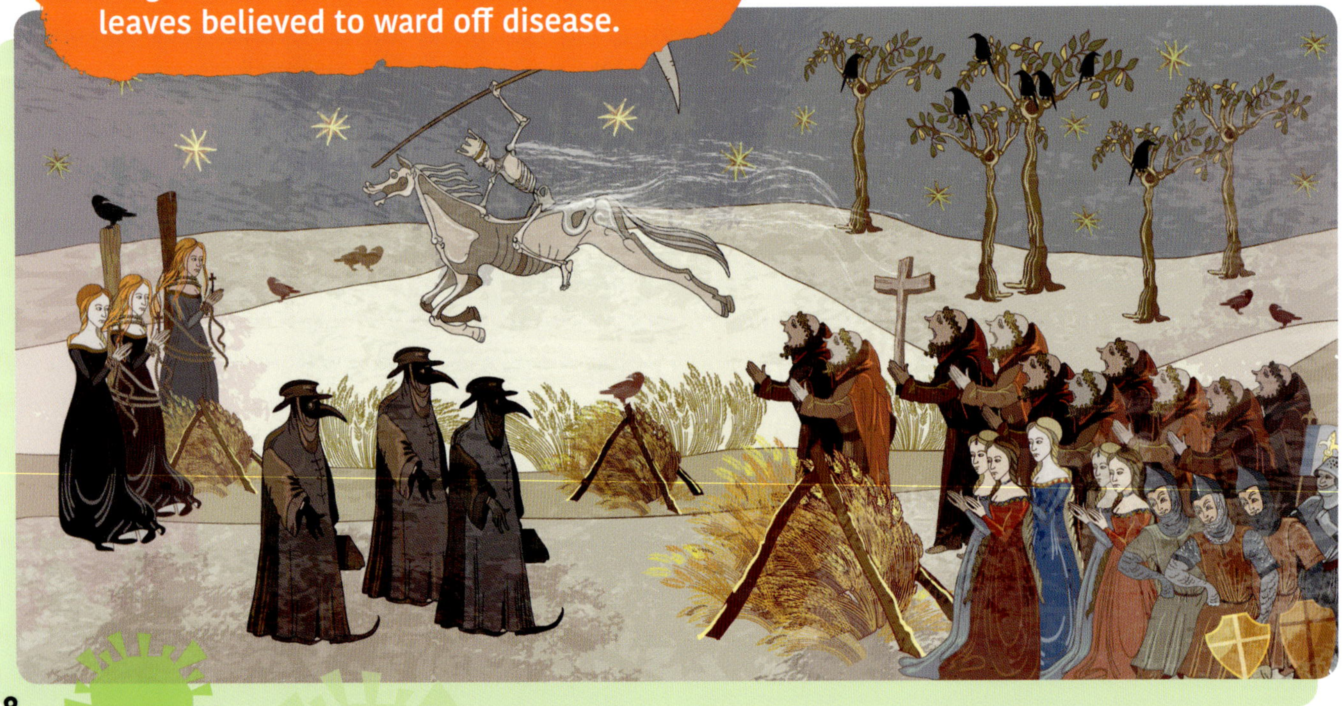

THROUGHOUT HISTORY

PANDEMIC HERO

Dr. Edward Jenner

Dr. Edward Jenner lived during a time when there were few effective treatments for many common diseases. Dr. Jenner's keen observations and determined scientific work helped eliminate the deadly smallpox virus. It also laid the foundation for modern **vaccines**. In the 1700s, smallpox outbreaks regularly killed and scarred thousands of people each year. But, mysteriously, English dairymaids seemed unharmed. Most of them had already been infected with a milder, related virus called cowpox. They had caught it through contact with infected dairy cows. Dr. Jenner believed that infecting people with cowpox on purpose could help protect them against smallpox. Because vaccines did not exist, he used a process called inoculation. This involved taking fresh cowpox pus from an infected person and inserting it into another person through a cut on their arm. In 1796, Dr. Jenner inoculated eight-year-old James Phipps using cowpox pus from Sarah Nelms, who milked cows. His experiment was initially rejected by other scientists but, over time, vaccinations became common. The last case of smallpox was recorded in 1977. This disease that was responsible for the deaths of hundreds of millions of people, was officially declared eradicated in 1980.

The Latin words for cow and cowpox are *vacca* and *vaccinia*. So, Jenner decided to name his new procedure "vaccination".

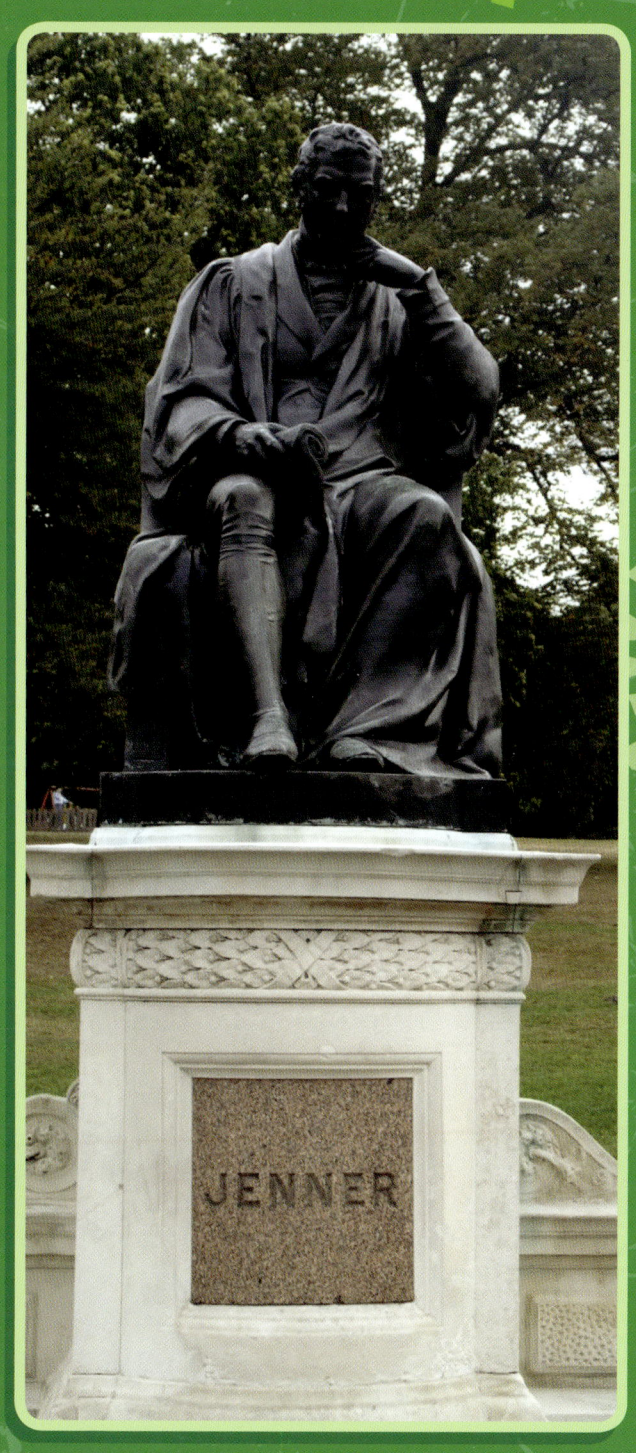

Chapter 1

Cities and Disease

Cities have played an important role in human development. They are busy places, with lots of people moving around from homes to schools and businesses. That makes them perfect breeding grounds for infectious diseases, which are **transmitted** from one person to the next.

Waste and Filth

In the past, cities often had open sewers, contaminated water supplies, and poor sanitation facilities. But many modern cities have well-established systems to provide clean water, waste removal, health services, and safe housing. This has had an impact on the health and life expectancy of city and country dwellers. People in modern cities, particularly in the **developed world**, live longer lives. They live two years longer, on average, than people in the country. In the past, it was quite the opposite.

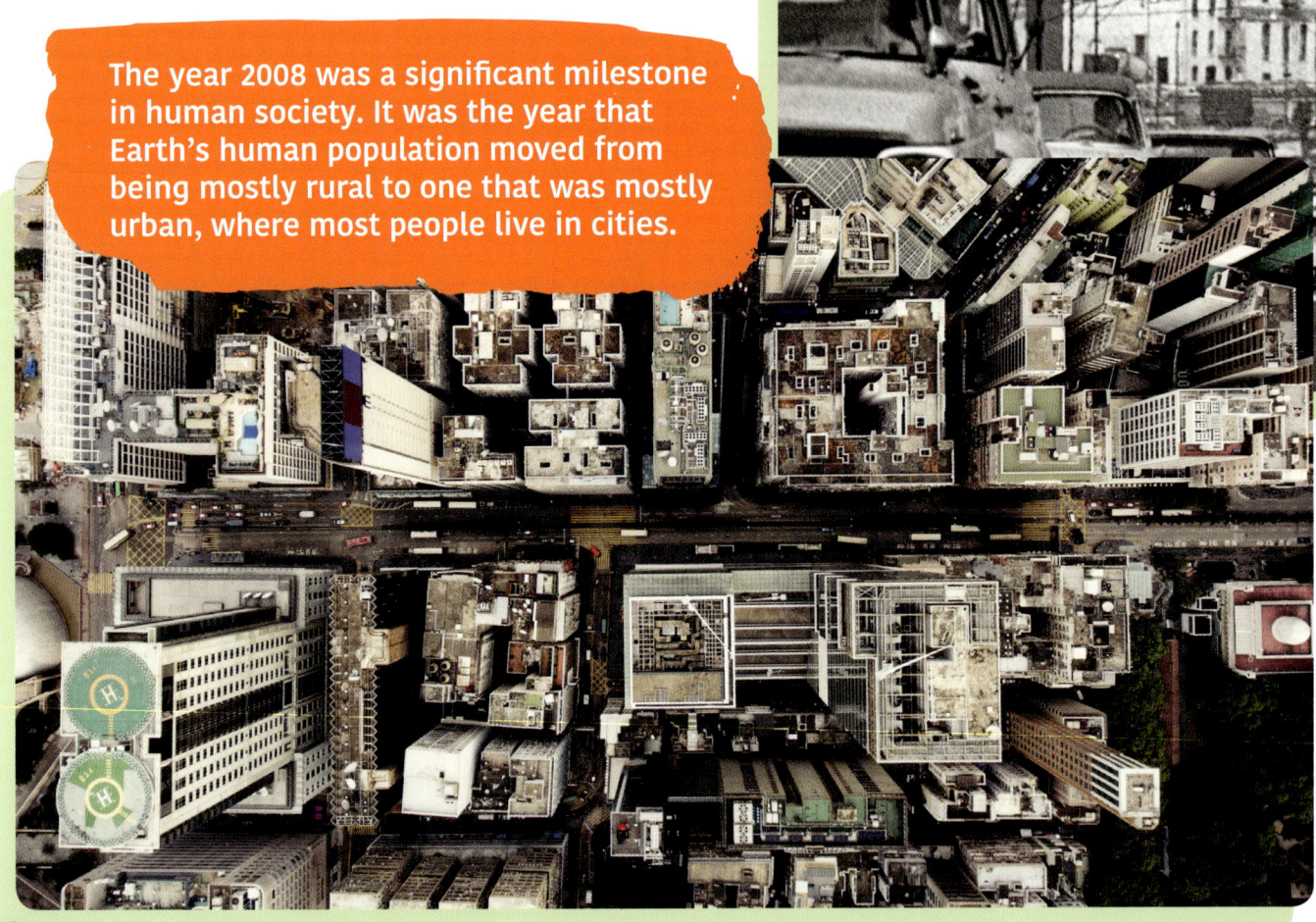

The year 2008 was a significant milestone in human society. It was the year that Earth's human population moved from being mostly rural to one that was mostly urban, where most people live in cities.

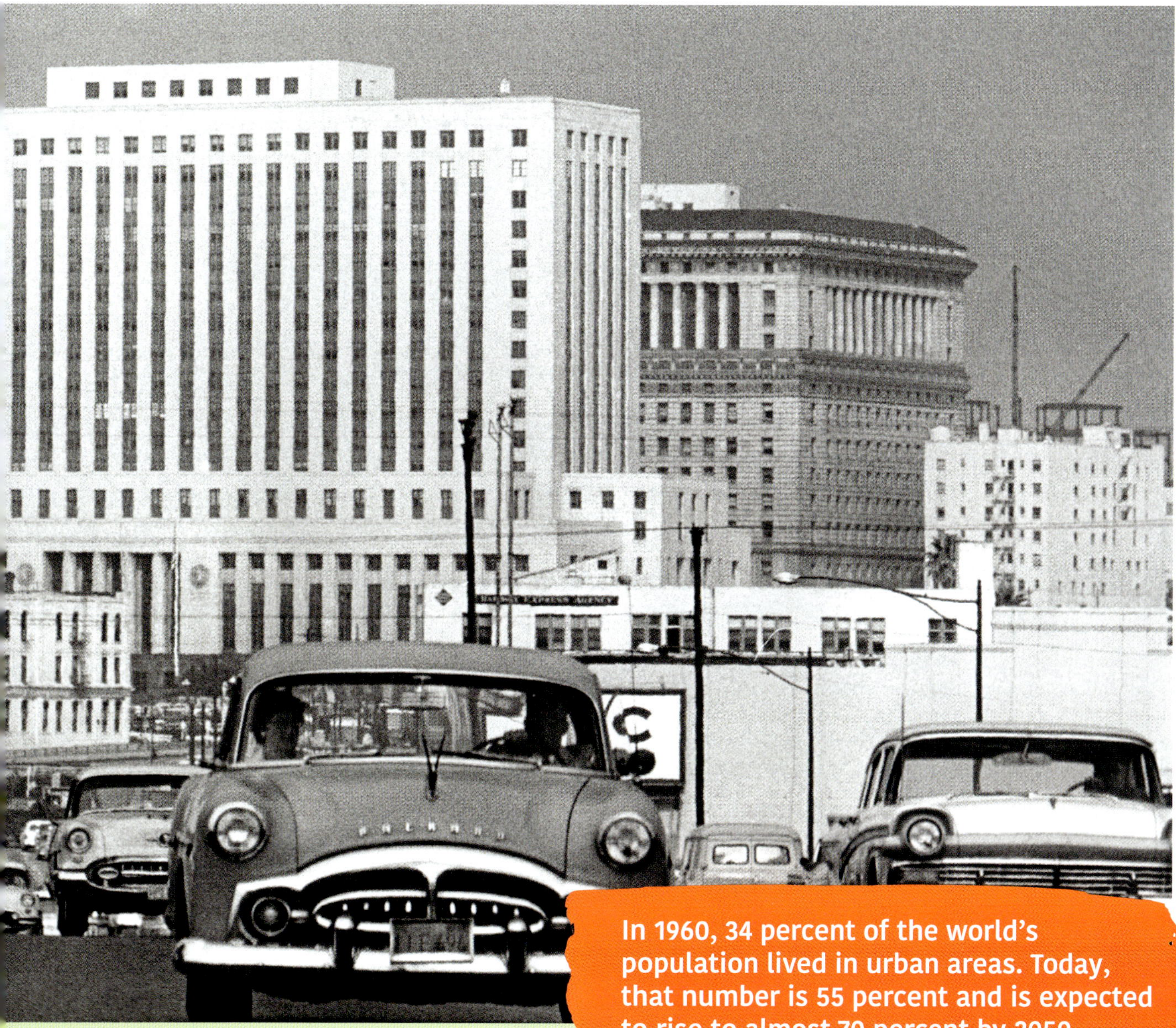

THROUGHOUT HISTORY

> In 1960, 34 percent of the world's population lived in urban areas. Today, that number is 55 percent and is expected to rise to almost 70 percent by 2050.

Urban Risks

For all their benefits, cities can also pose risks. The more **densely populated** a city is, where large numbers of people live closely together, the larger the risk of transmitting disease. This means the risk of pandemics is greater than ever. These pandemics can have serious consequences for all of us. They affect our health and safety, our livelihoods, food supplies, and global economies.

Scientists made great progress in developing vaccines to treat viruses that once killed millions. But new viruses have appeared during the last century and pose new threats. As our cities continue to expand in size, they are **encroaching** on wild animal habitats. As contact between the two increases, so does the likelihood of disease transmission from animals to humans.

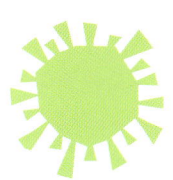

Chapter 1

Ebola is a conservation threat to great apes such as gorillas and chimpanzees. This means these animals get sick and die from the disease. It can also be passed on to humans who eat bush meat. The meat from these animals is not properly prepared. As the forests these animals live in are cut down, there is more chance of human contact and more chance of the disease spreading to humans.

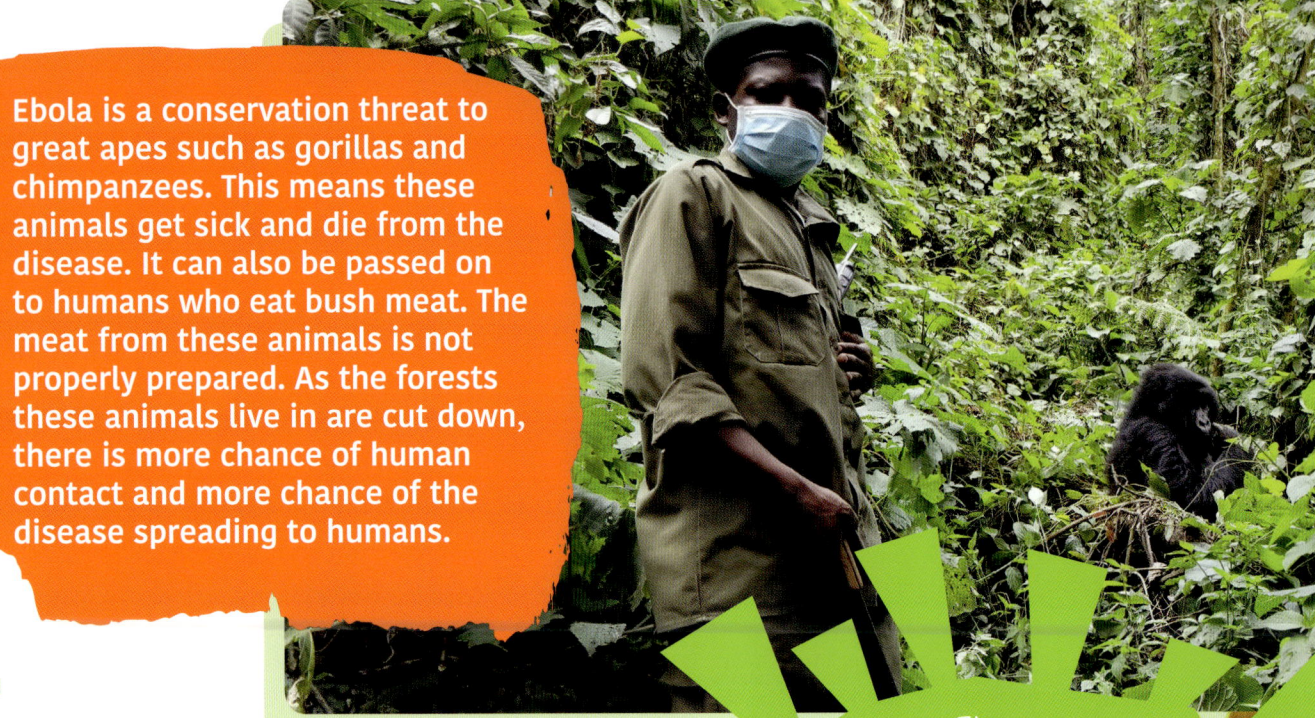

Some people worry that new diseases are becoming more frequent. What we learn from each new outbreak can help us learn how to avoid future pandemics.

Ebola

As populations grow and cities expand, humans are coming in closer contact with wildlife. Ebola was first discovered in 1976. It is a virus that causes a severe fever and bleeding. It was transmitted from infected fruit bats, chimps, and gorillas to humans. To reduce the likelihood of disease transmission in the future, scientists are working to better understand how viruses cross over between species.

Ebola is a viral hemorrhagic fever. This means blood hemorrhages, or escapes abnormally, from the circulatory system. This causes internal bleeding in the body and external bleeding from eyes, nose, and mouth. Ebola is spread through direct contact with the bodily fluids of infected people. It is very contagious.

SARS

A disease called Severe Acute Respiratory Syndrome, or SARS, appeared in China in 2003. Delays in sharing information between health systems and governments allowed SARS to spread quickly. Governments were slow to set up quarantine. To quarantine is to keep people who have a disease separate from those who do not. This slow action caused many unnecessary deaths. It became clear that information must be shared openly, honestly, and swiftly between countries to effectively fight disease outbreaks.

MERS

Middle East Respiratory Syndrome (MERS) is a virus that affects the respiratory system, or lungs. When a citizen in South Korea developed flu-like symptoms in 2015, there was little information available from the **World Health Organization (WHO)**. As the number of cases rose, people were unaware of how it was spreading and who was infected. The rollout of testing was slow. People lost trust in their government to protect them. Finally, a national testing program was developed to identify and track the outbreak.

CORONAVIRUSES

Like COVID-19, SARS and MERS are caused by coronaviruses. Coronaviruses are a large family of viruses. Most affect animals, meaning they are zoonotic. Some have jumped from animals to humans. Over the past 20 years, three of these have caused serious illnesses and death. Those illnesses are SARS, MERS, and COVID-19. Researchers have been studying ways to prevent more zoonotic diseases from emerging.

> It is believed that MERS first infected bats. However, humans were infected from close contact with camels.

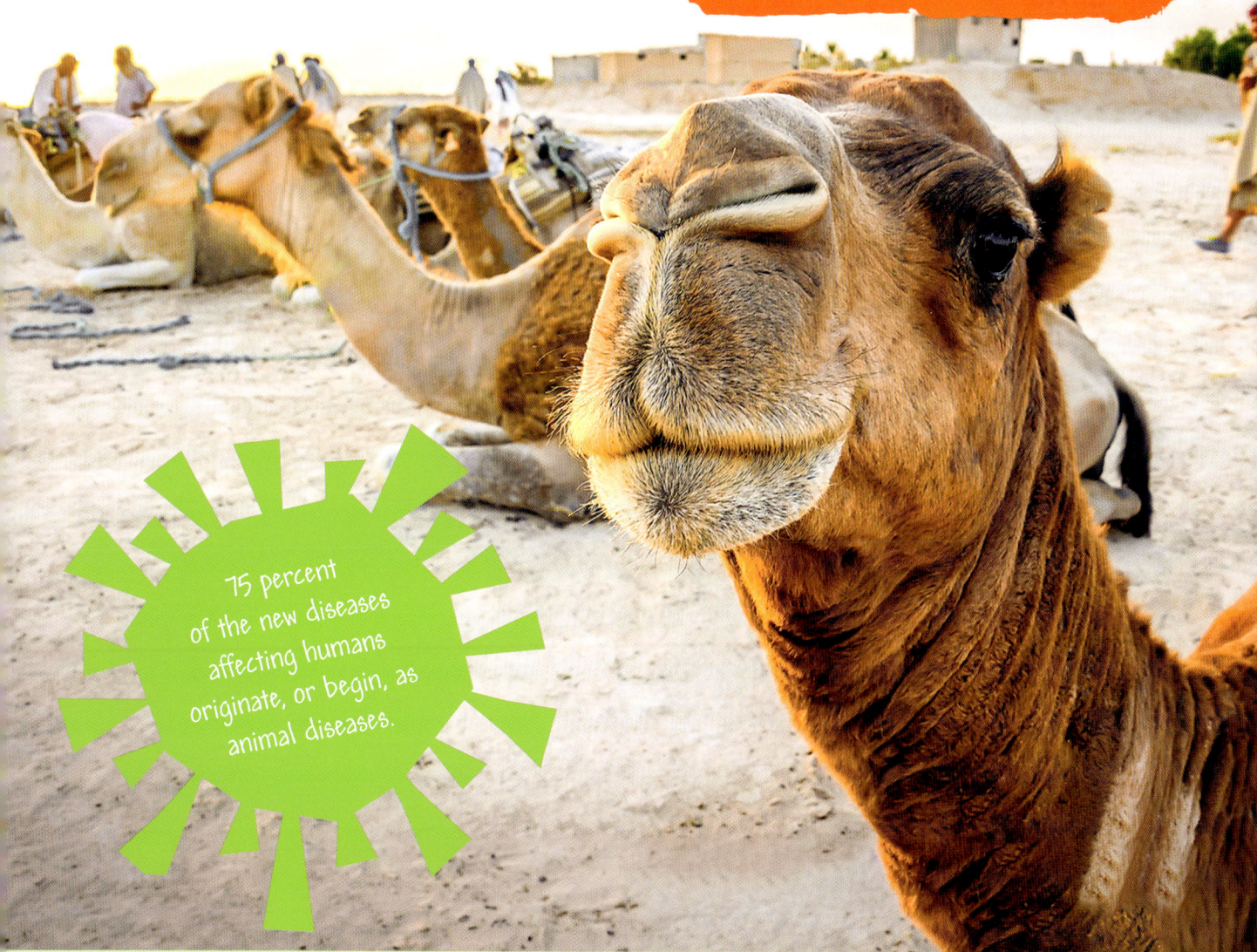

75 percent of the new diseases affecting humans originate, or begin, as animal diseases.

Chapter 2

The COVID-19 Pandemic

While the world watched, more and more people fell ill in China. The virus continued its stealthy spread across the planet. Travelers carried it across international borders to an unsuspecting and unprepared world. By the time people began to really understand what was happening, the virus was already in Europe and the Middle East. Within weeks, it had spread around the world.

Few infectious disease experts were surprised by the arrival of a new pandemic. In fact, many had been sounding the alarm for years. In today's connected world, humans and animals are in increasingly closer contact. It is a perfect breeding ground for infectious diseases.

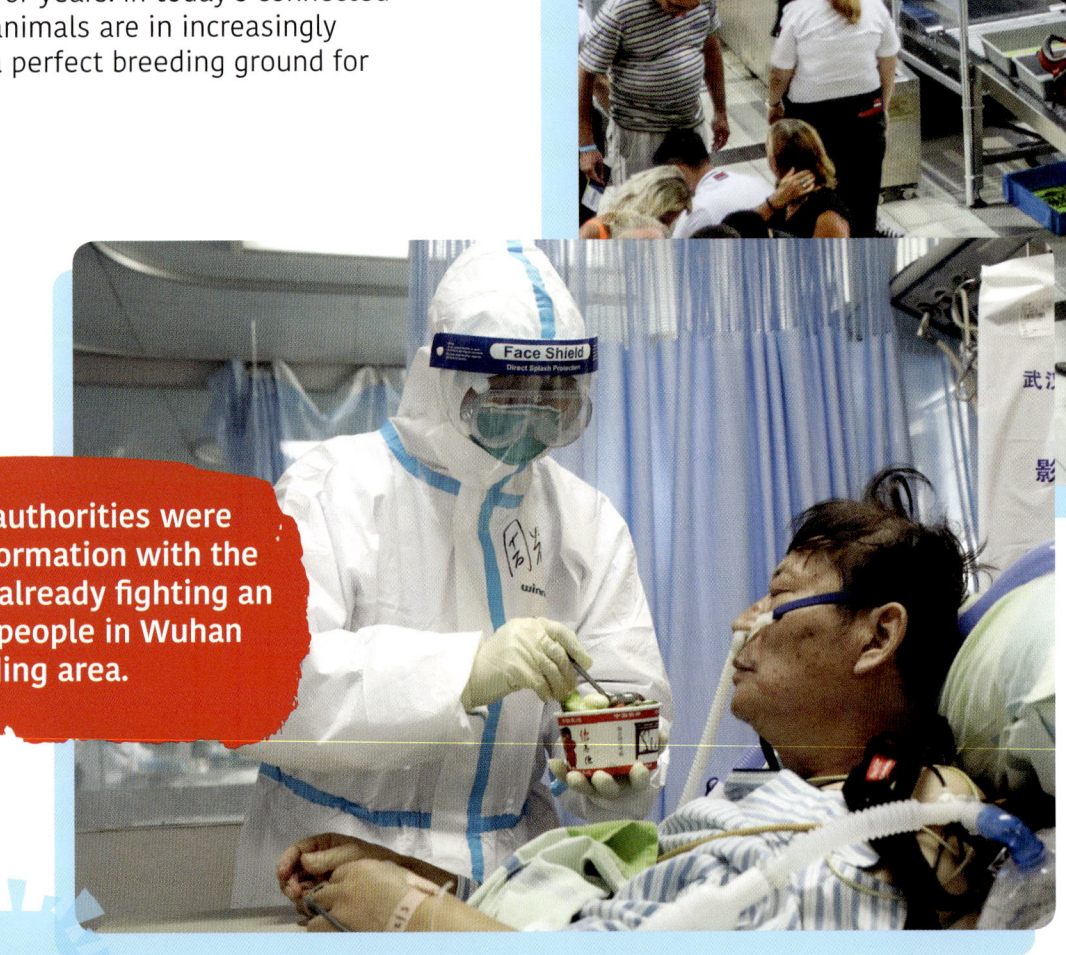

At first, Chinese authorities were slow to share information with the WHO. They were already fighting an epidemic of sick people in Wuhan and the surrounding area.

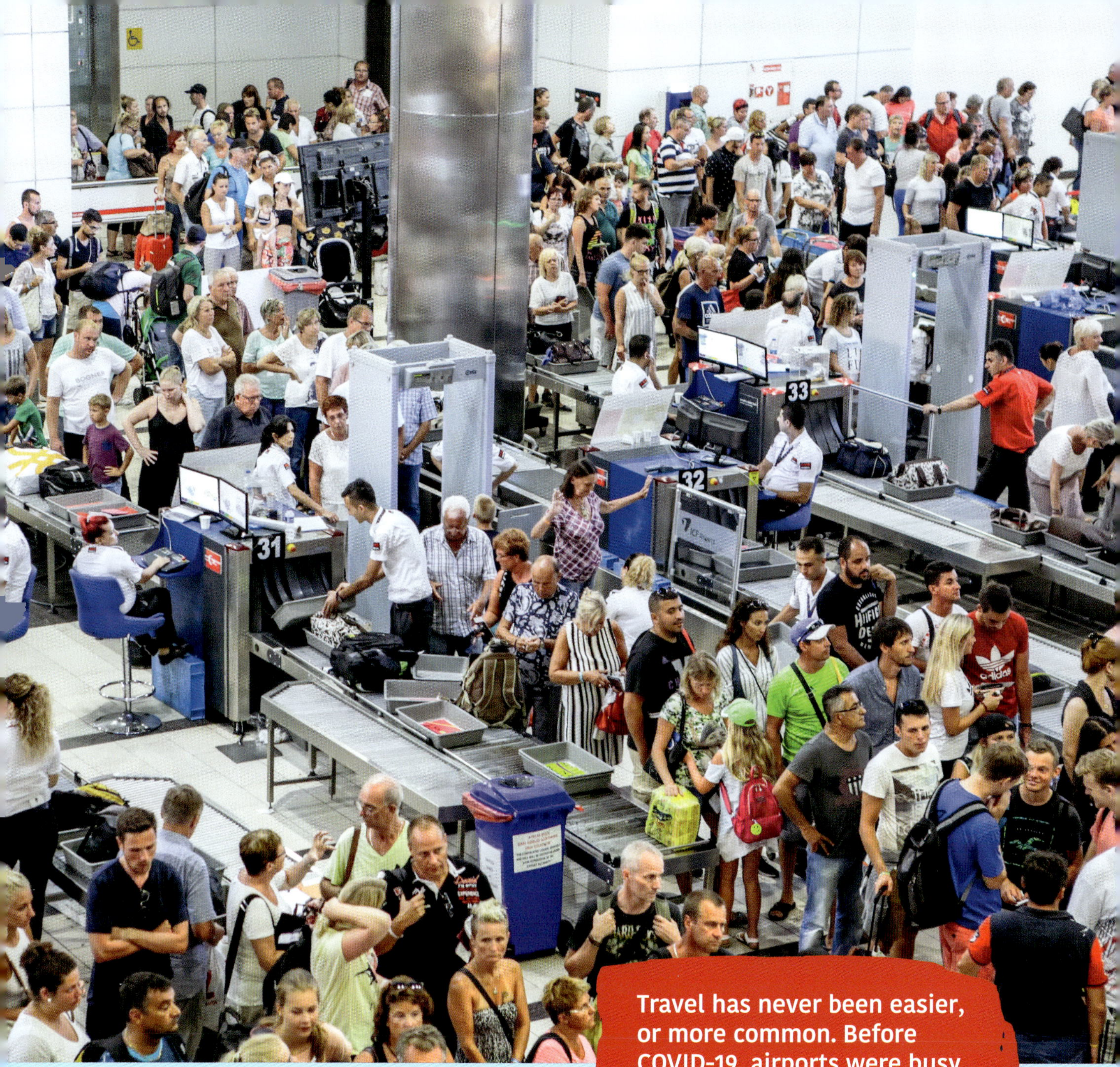

Travel has never been easier, or more common. Before COVID-19, airports were busy with people traveling all over the world. Experts now know the virus that causes COVID-19 spread throughout the world before we knew it existed.

Ignoring the Risks

Despite warnings about new pandemics, many governments have continued to ignore the risks. Public health organizations work to develop programs that would help prevent, identify, and control future outbreaks. But they have been poorly funded, or provided with money, by governments. The reluctance to share information in the early days of the COVID-19 outbreak suggests that there is still a lack of trust between countries. This continues to put eveyone in danger.

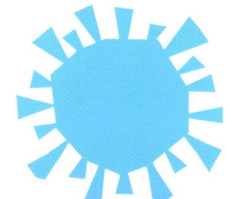

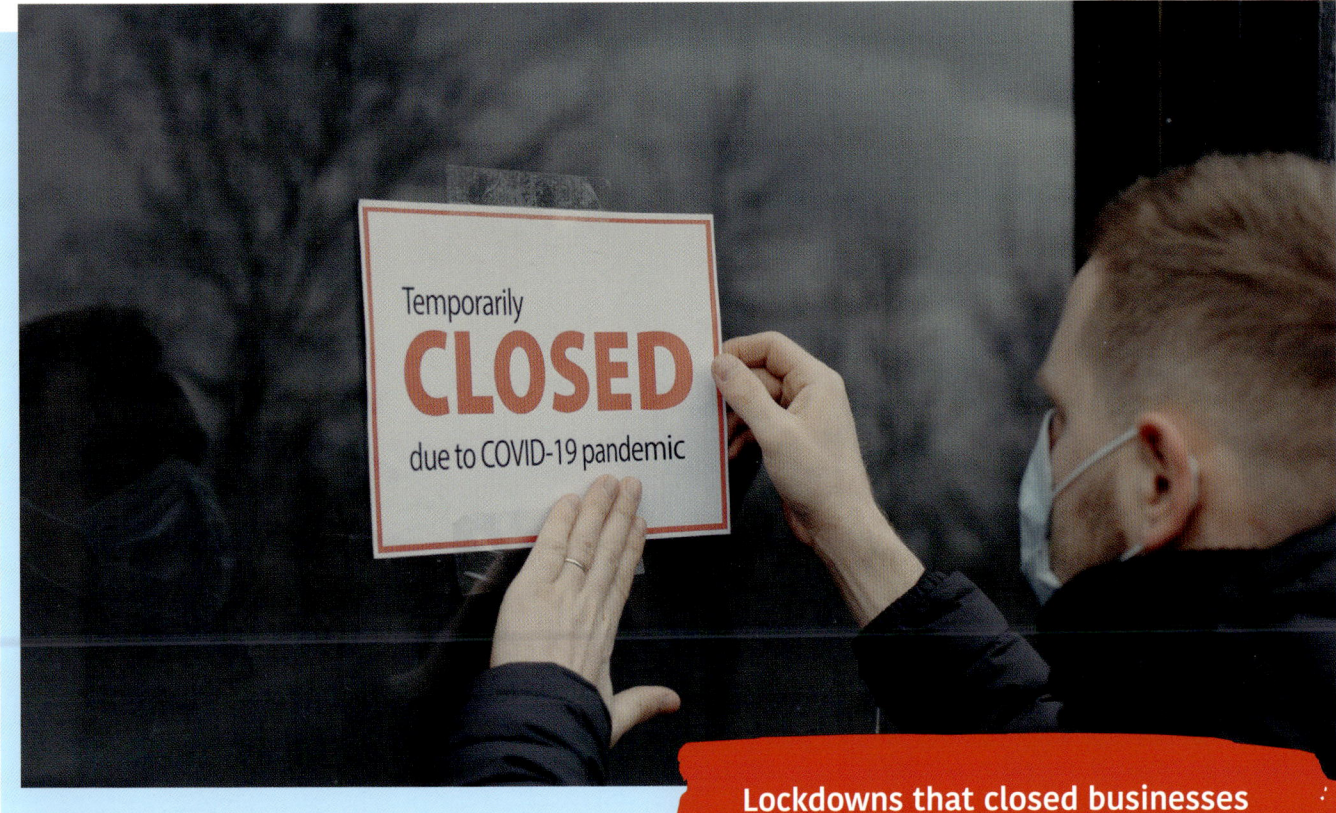

Lockdowns that closed businesses and schools were one method that governments used to protect people.

Slowing a Deadly Pandemic

While some governments were slow to react, others denied that the situation was serious. By the time public health measures were enacted, hundreds of thousands of people all over the world were infected and the virus began to spread more quickly. The disease spread easily in populated areas such as cities. Soon, governments were forced to take extreme measures to respond to the crisis.

Stay At Home

Public spaces were restricted, and "stay-at-home" orders were issued. **Nonessential** businesses were forced to close. People were encouraged to work from home. Schools shut down, forcing students to take classes online. Many borders closed and nonessential travel was discouraged, but not prevented. Frontline workers, such as grocery store workers, truck drivers, and health care providers, became heroes. They provided the services necessary to save lives and keep cities functioning.

Limited Freedom

While these steps helped save lives, they also had downsides. The ability to move freely was restricted. People could not shop, travel, socialize, and be entertained in the usual ways. Many people's mental health suffered as families and friends were isolated from one another. Hospitals and medical staff were stressed by the numbers of sick people being treated. Businesses were hard hit. Many small businesses closed permanently, causing people to lose jobs, homes, and security. The impact on city and community ways of life was devastating. The economies of entire countries were affected.

PANDEMIC HERO

Alanna Badgley

Alanna Badgley knows how important a single breath can be. It's the first thing we do when we're born and the last before we die. As a paramedic in Westchester County, New York, she has seen how difficult a single breath can be for people infected with COVID-19. Badgley arose most mornings before sunrise to pack her medical kit and prepare for the day. By the time she had finished her shift 12 hours later, she had often responded to more than 10 emergency calls. COVID-19 patients often died alone, with their families unable to visit, hold their hands, or say goodbye. So, Alanna did her best to take their families' place—holding patients' hands and sharing comforting and encouraging words. Alanna was one of hundreds of thousands of health care workers around the world who risked their lives to help others.

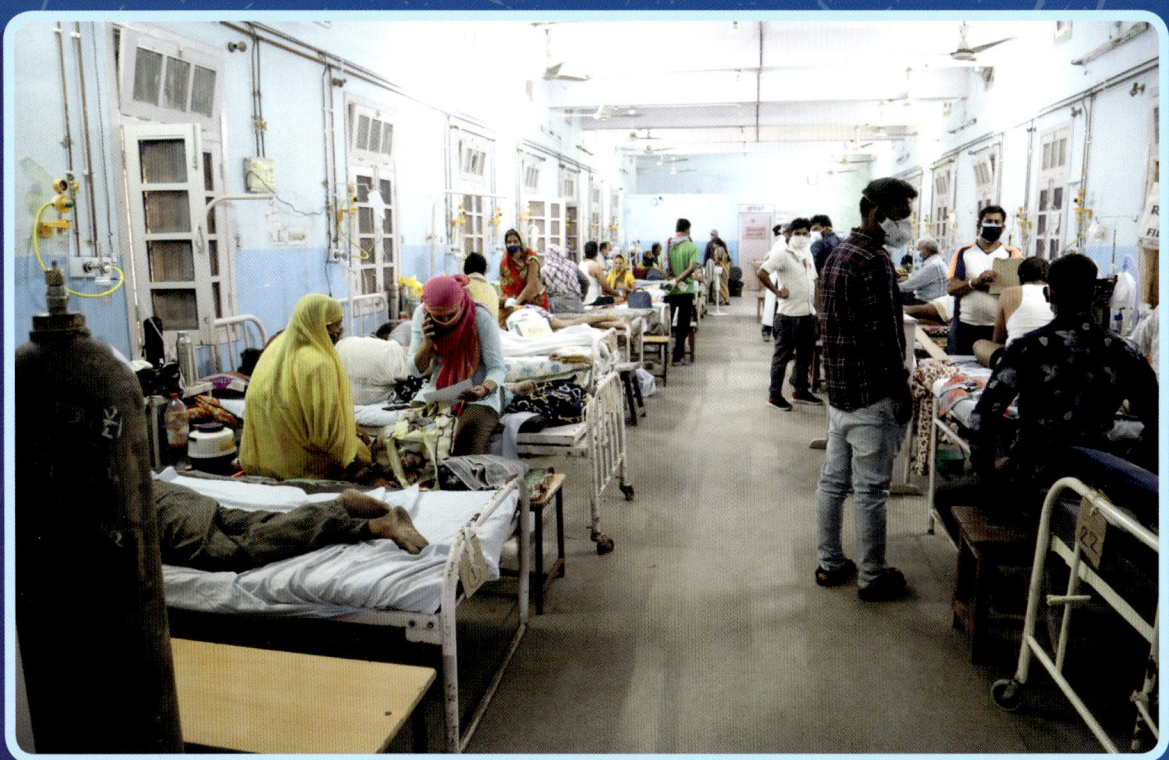

When hospitals in bigger cities overflowed with patients, sick people were sent to hospitals in smaller communities. In India in May 2021, families searched for hospitals that had enough beds and often bought their own oxygen tanks. In some cases, family members cared for their loved ones themselves because there were not enough nurses and doctors.

Chapter 2

How Cities Coped with COVID-19

As cities across the globe responded to the COVID-19 pandemic, they did so in very different ways. Wuhan, China, with a population of 11 million, was the first city to confront the virus. Government restrictions were among the strictest in the world. The city was under a total lockdown for many months until the virus was under control. People's movements were strictly monitored by police and security. Punishments for rule-breakers were harsh. Ten months and 4,000 deaths later, the city began to return to normal.

Seoul, Korea

Seoul, South Korea, used the lessons it learned from an earlier epidemic to guide its response to COVID-19. Its strategy relied on three ideas: fast and free testing, strong tracing technology, and mandatory isolation. This allowed Koreans to limit the spread of the virus without stay-at-home orders. In the **first wave**, Seoul counted less than 100 deaths in a city of 9 million people. It wasn't until the fourth wave in 2021, that the country added widespread closures.

Johannesburg, South Africa

Johannesburg, South Africa, is a city of contrasts. There is great wealth and great **inequality**. Like most other African countries, South Africa imposed a national lockdown early in the pandemic. It used community contact tracing teams that were established for **tuberculosis** control. They monitored and traced people who tested positive. Almost 11.2 million people, or 20 percent of the population, were screened early on. But continued testing and finding enough personal protective equipment (PPE) was difficult. This, combined with dense population in poor areas, led to the virus spreading. As a result, South Africa had among the highest numbers of infections in the world in the first wave.

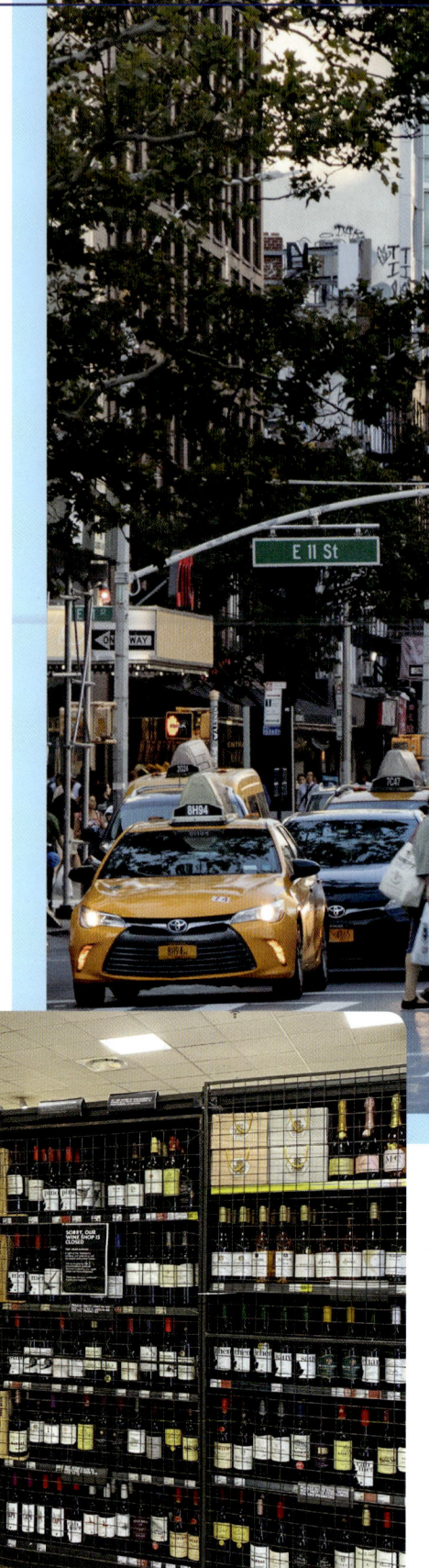

The South African government imposed a nightly **curfew** and alcohol ban to help slow the spread of the virus. These were lifted when the economy began to fail.

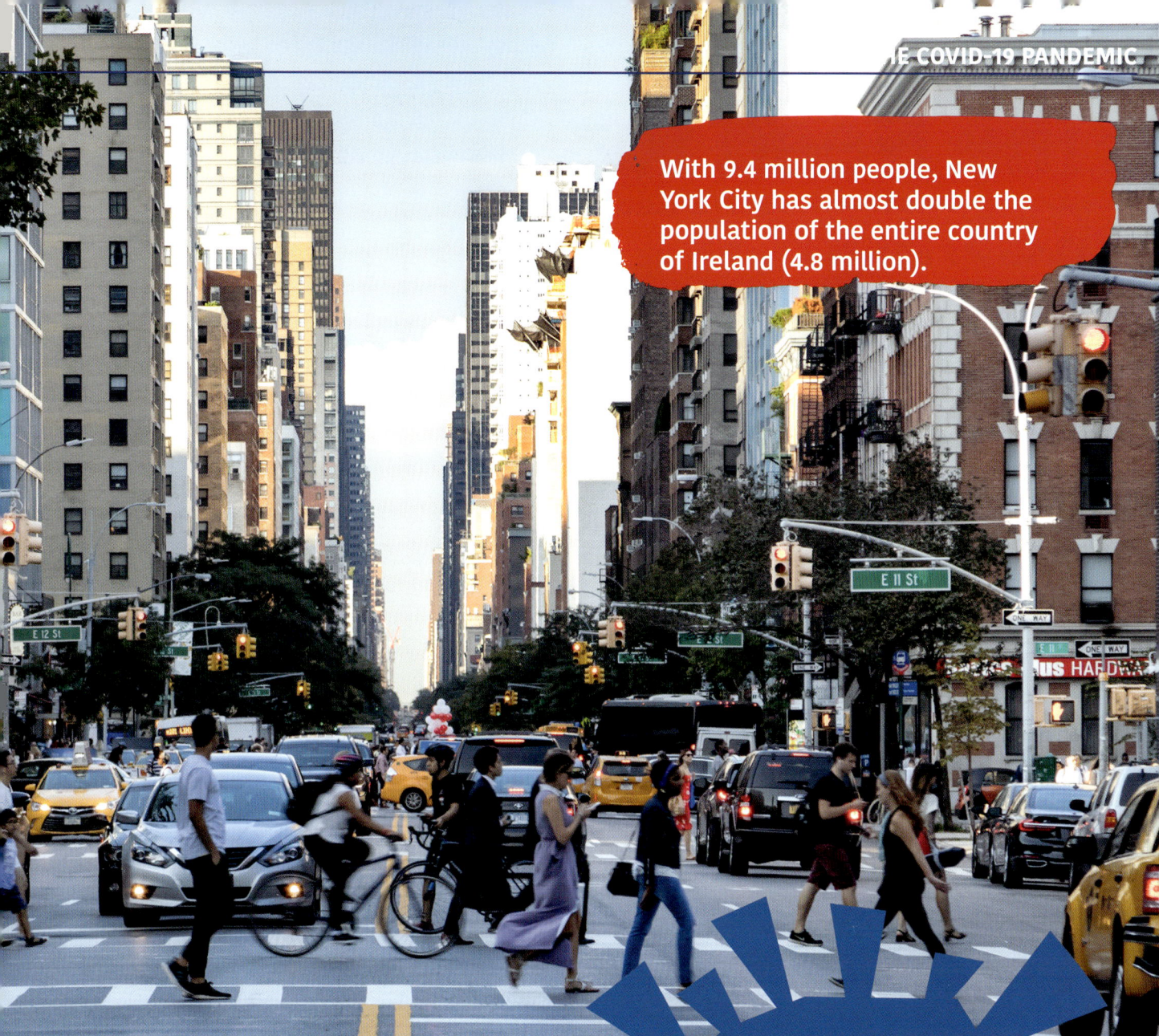

With 9.4 million people, New York City has almost double the population of the entire country of Ireland (4.8 million).

New York City

In the first wave of COVID-19, New York City struggled to keep up with the numbers of sick and dying. With little testing at first and almost no personal restrictions in place, the virus spread uncontrollably for weeks. By the time a stay-at-home order was issued for the state of New York on March 20, 2020, infections were high. Hospitals were quickly overwhelmed and forced to **ration** PPE. This put medical staff in danger. More than 19,000 people died in the first wave, making it one of the worst-hit cities anywhere.

New York City used 85 refrigerated trailers to hold the bodies of the dead during the first wave. Morgues and cemeteries could not handle the numbers. In April 2020, up to 800 people died per day.

Chapter 3

The Need for Resilience

During the past century, many cities have grown dramatically. As a result, billions of dollars have been spent to create better infrastructure. Infrastructure includes the roads, public transit, hospitals, safe water supplies, and sanitation services that make living in a city safe. A community's livability is measured on its ability to provide citizens with the things they need to live healthy, productive, and long lives.

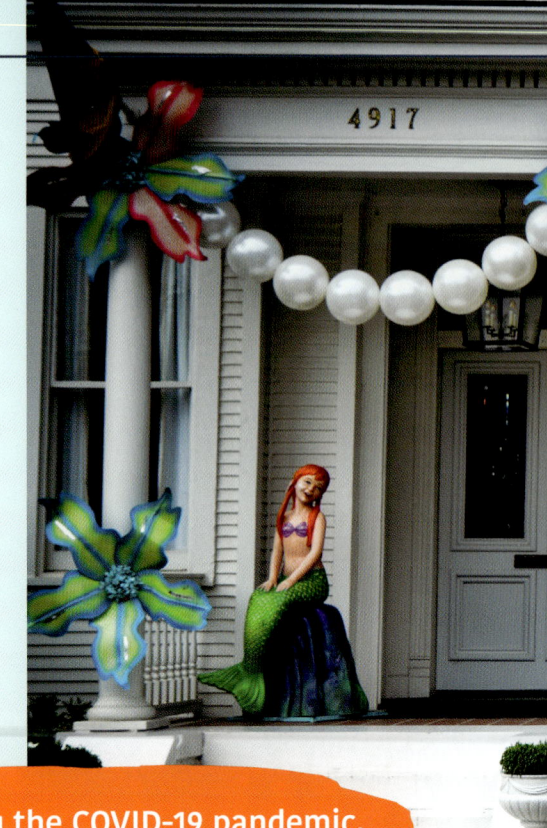

What Is Resilience?

Many communities are working on building resilience. Resilience means the ability to adapt to change and recover from economic, environmental, or social setbacks. Economic setbacks may mean a lot of businesses that have closed leaving people unemployed. Environmental setbacks might mean severe weather, such as hurricanes or tornadoes, that destroy buildings and damage infrastructure. Social setbacks may mean the interruption of people's normal ways of living. Communities that are resilient can respond to crises and can keep citizens safe with few disruptions to their daily lives.

> During the COVID-19 pandemic, people could no longer gather in big groups. In 2021, the city of New Orleans, Louisiana, canceled its famous Mardi Gras carnival after the 2020 parades and gatherings proved to be virus spreaders. Instead, people decorated their homes so others could view them from a distance.

Pandemics and Change

Pandemics are a special challenge for cities. They impact how cities and communities function economically, environmentally, and socially. As cities grow, they become more densely populated. Many large buildings house thousands of people. There is less room to social distance in private and public spaces. This means that there is a greater opportunity for diseases to spread.

During COVID-19, many cities found that the pandemic challenged the normal way of life. In New York City, more people were working from home, so fewer people used public transit. But the transit system still needed to function for people who did travel to jobs. Now the transit system needs to deal with the reality that ridership may never be the same, but it still needs money to run.

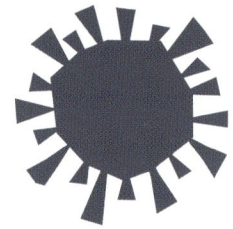

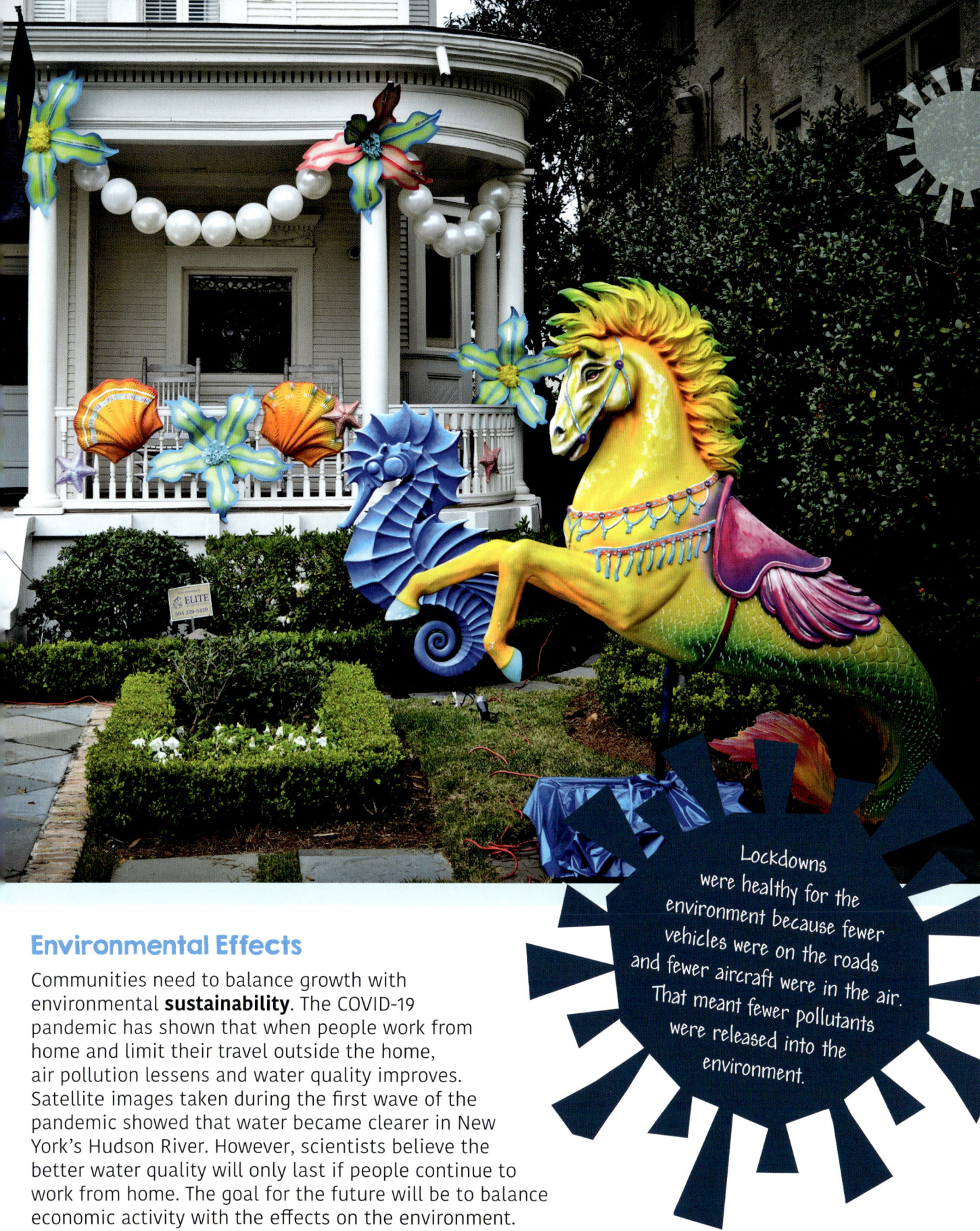

Environmental Effects

Communities need to balance growth with environmental **sustainability**. The COVID-19 pandemic has shown that when people work from home and limit their travel outside the home, air pollution lessens and water quality improves. Satellite images taken during the first wave of the pandemic showed that water became clearer in New York's Hudson River. However, scientists believe the better water quality will only last if people continue to work from home. The goal for the future will be to balance economic activity with the effects on the environment.

Lockdowns were healthy for the environment because fewer vehicles were on the roads and fewer aircraft were in the air. That meant fewer pollutants were released into the environment.

Chapter 3

Most at Risk

The virus did not affect everyone the same. People who were able to isolate and work from home were less likely to contract the virus. Workplace transmission was significant among essential workers. These included health care workers, construction, and factory and food service workers. In the United States, COVID-19 had a **disproportionate** impact on Black and Latinx people. This was because many work in frontline jobs. Those workers also brought the virus home—meaning their communities were also at greater risk.

Homelessness and COVID-19

In many communities, some groups of people—including the **unhoused** and disabled—have less access to services. It is difficult for unhoused people to isolate and remain distant, especially if they are living in shelters. The disabled depend on services that may be interrupted during lockdowns. Protecting all citizens during a pandemic is as important as stopping the spread of a disease.

> COVID-19 showed that people who lived in crowded housing and worked in jobs where they could not be 6 feet (2 m) apart from others were more likely to contract the virus.

THE NEED FOR RESILIENCE

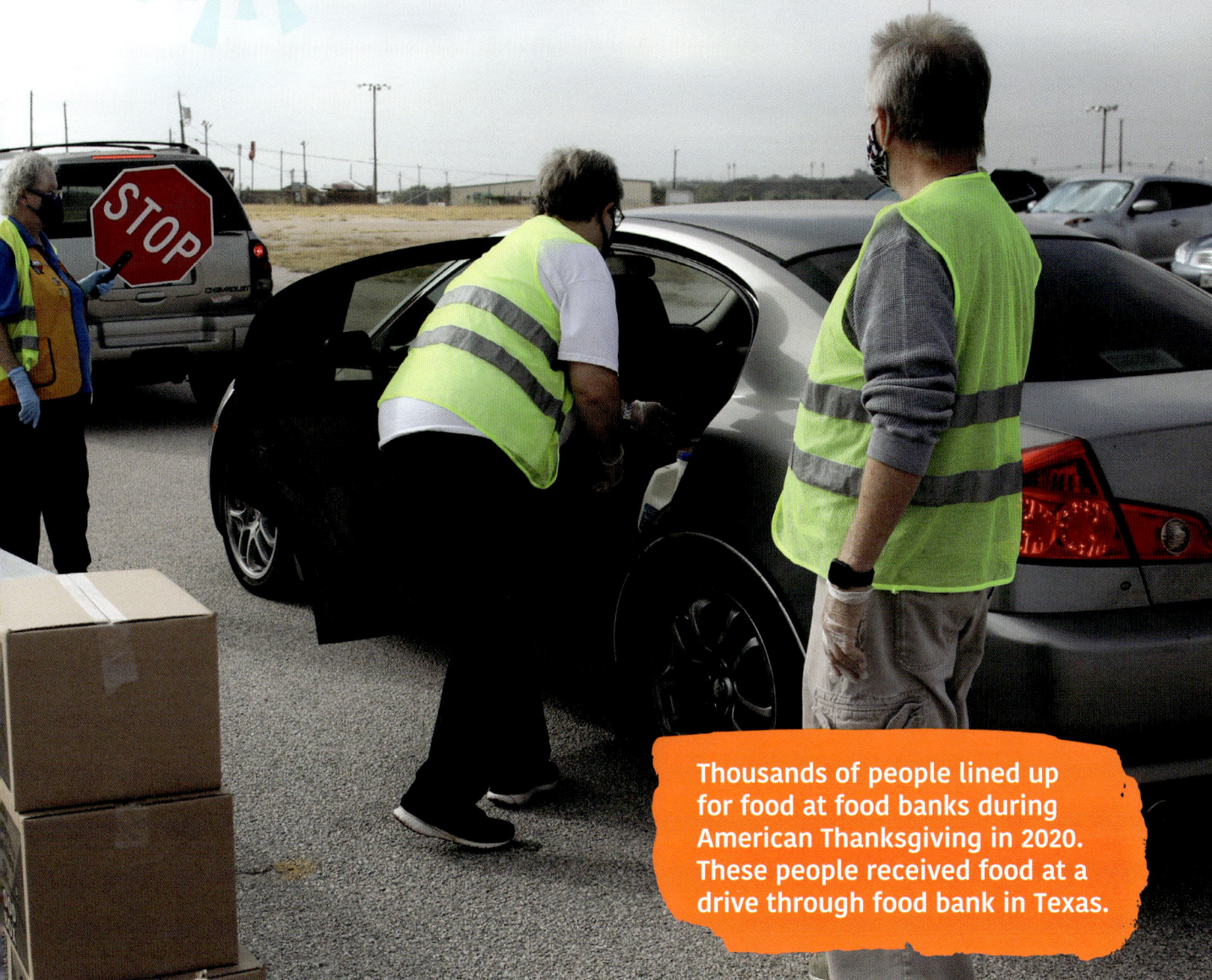

Thousands of people lined up for food at food banks during American Thanksgiving in 2020. These people received food at a drive through food bank in Texas.

Elderly and Isolation

The elderly, the poor, and the disabled are **vulnerable** populations. That means they are normally at greater risk of poor health. They are also more likely to be isolated with fewer supports. During the COVID-19 pandemic, those vulnerabilities were made worse. Those groups had higher transmission rates. Their mental health suffered as well, because the stress of living day-to-day with little support wore many people down. Resilient communities would provide these groups with easier access to medical care and personal support, and the ability to move around their community safely.

Working Hard During COVID

Many lower-paid workers rely on multiple part-time or short-term jobs for their income. During a pandemic, these groups are much more likely to lose one or more of their jobs. Job losses made poverty worse during COVID-19. More people had to rely on food banks for groceries. According to the food bank network Feeding America, more than 80 percent of the country's food banks were serving more people during COVID-19 than they did the year before the pandemic. An estimated one in six Americans faced hunger because of the pandemic.

Chapter 3

What is a Resilient City?

Resilient cities help people and businesses adapt and thrive no matter what difficulties they face. These cities not only provide basic services such as safe water, housing, health care, education, and jobs, but they are also prepared for crises. They can respond effectively when faced with sudden emergencies such as severe storms, earthquakes, floods, or pandemics. The reason they can do this is because they have planned for the future. These plans include the services they offer and the way the city is built.

Planned Resilience

Modern cities have planning departments with urban planners. They develop plans for how to use the land and resources such as water or forests. They work with others, such as builders, politicians, businesses, schools, and members of the public, to decide how a city should grow. The ideas of urban sustainability and resilience are not new. Modern cities have been trying to adapt to and survive changes and emergencies for many years. One way they do this is by developing a resilience strategy.

Resilience Strategy

Resilience strategies are plans that are made with the help of city residents. They examine a city's strengths and weaknesses, and come up with improvements based on what the residents feel is needed. The strategies also must fit with the city's overall plan for the future. To make a resilience strategy, residents and community groups may be asked by the city to answer simple **questionnaires**. They may also voice their opinions at special meetings. These opinions are studied and solutions are suggested. Each resilience strategy reflects the city's specific challenges or areas for improvement. One city may want to make housing more affordable. Another may want to improve public transit, making it easier for everyone to move around the city.

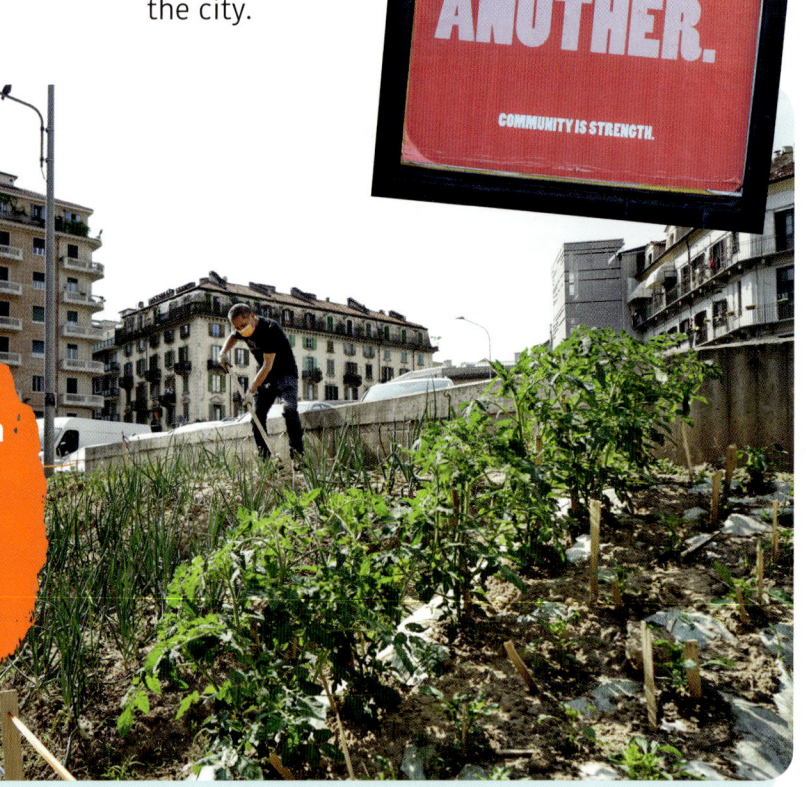

Resilience strategies require politicians and leaders to work with communities on what matters to their residents. One solution could be to establish community gardens in urban areas.

THE NEED FOR RESILIENCE

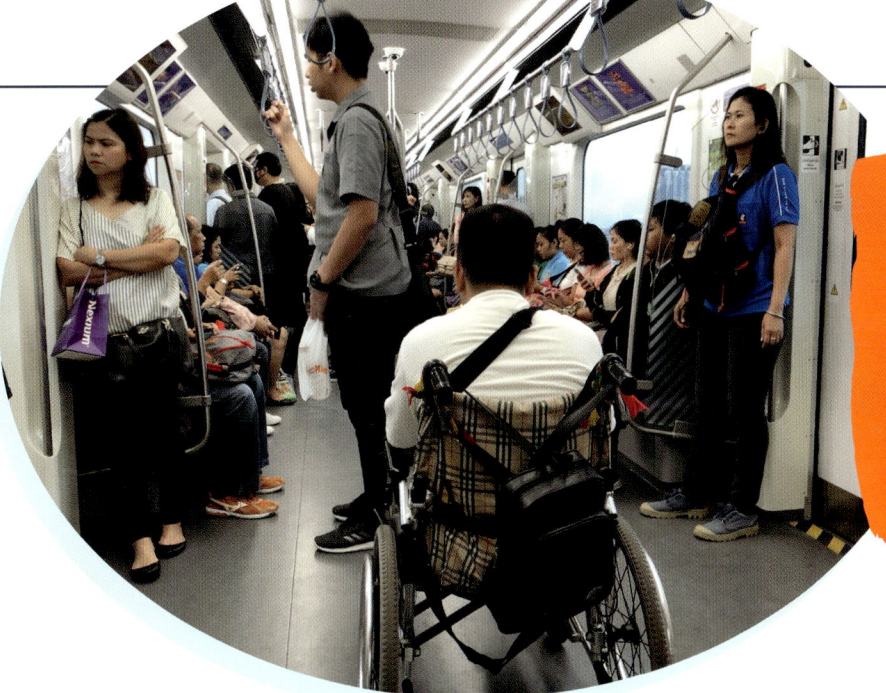

Public transit is important to city residents—especially during events such as pandemics. Making public transit safer, easier to access, and more affordable is one challenge for resilient cities.

PANDEMIC WHO'S WHO

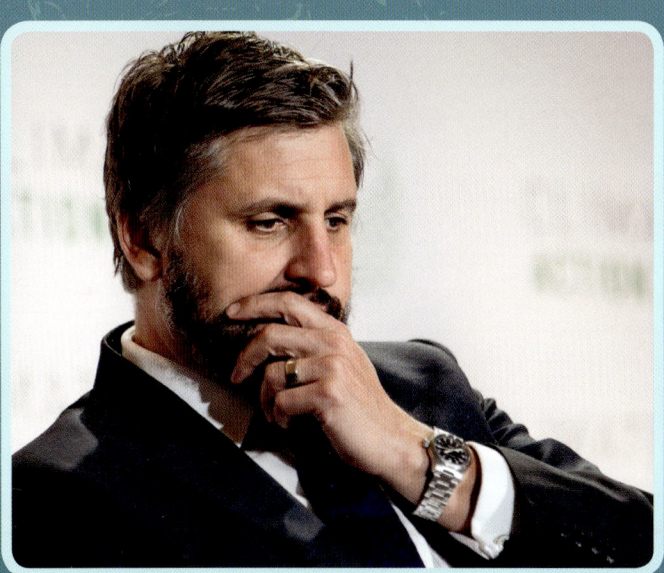

Berkowitz believes reinventing cities should be based on community-building ideas. These include getting to know neighbors and planting more trees to make streets greener and more pedestrian-friendly.

Michael Berkowitz

Michael Berkowitz spends a lot of time thinking about disasters. For much of his career, he has worked with governments around the world to help plan for hurricanes and disease outbreaks. As the COVID-19 pandemic raged across the world, he was passionate about finding ways to help strengthen the resilience of cities and countries. Michael is one of the founders of the Resilient Cities Catalyst. This is a **nonprofit** organization that helps cities tackle disasters. He believes cities will need to resist the temptation to simply rebuild and replace what was there before. Berkowitz thinks it is smarter to reinvent cities and communities to make them better places to live.

Chapter 4

Resilience Strategies

Even before COVID-19 turned the world upside down, experts warned that we needed to make our communities more resilient so they could withstand disasters. In 2010, the United Nations Office for Disaster Risk Reduction created the Making Cities Resilient campaign to help cities cope with disasters.

Many cities have begun to develop creative strategies for survival and growth. But few have put a lot of effort into preparing for and protecting cities from global disease outbreaks. Long before COVID-19, **virologists** had been sounding the alarm that the next pandemic was just a matter of time. They knew that without systems in place to make the pandemic less severe, economies would be harmed. The Making Cities Resilient (MCR) campaign was launched to raise awareness of disaster risk and reduction. More than 4,300 cities around the world joined the project.

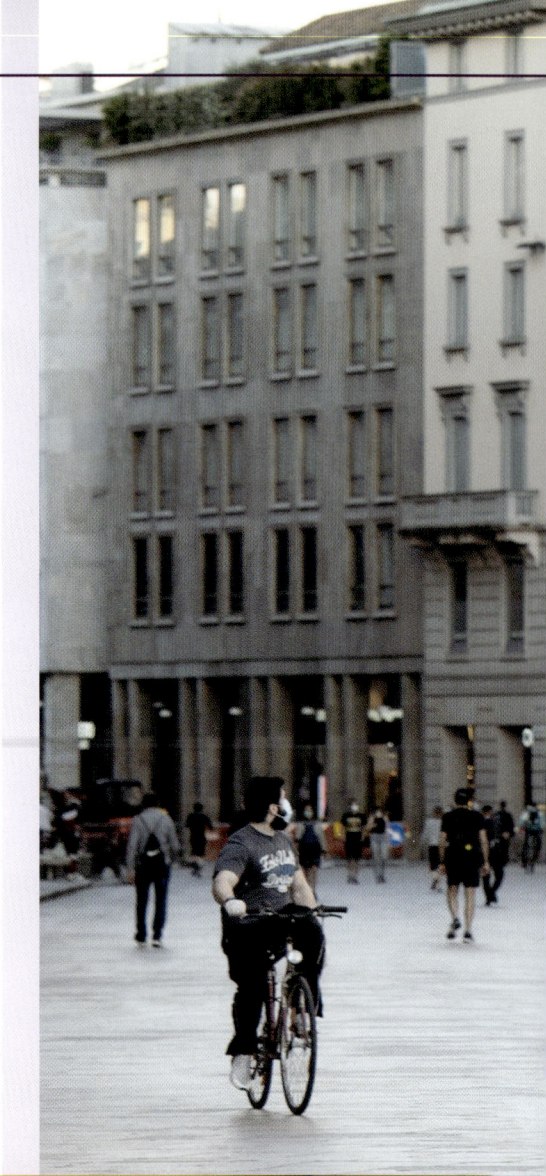

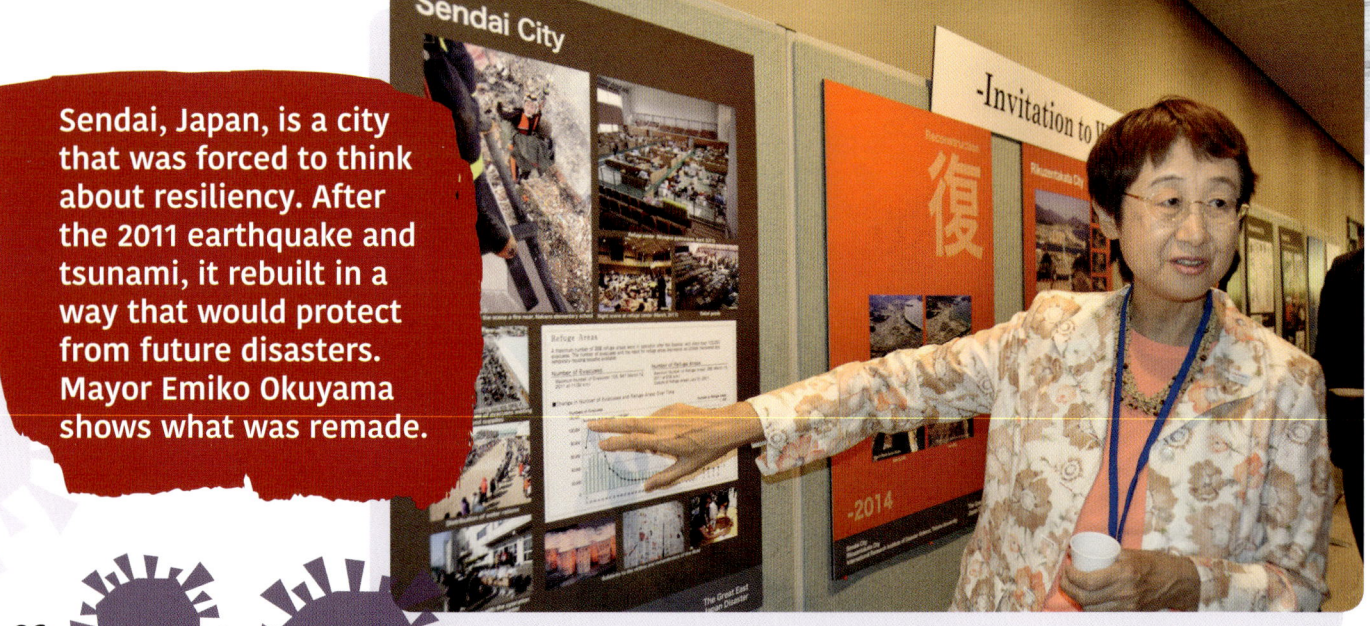

Sendai, Japan, is a city that was forced to think about resiliency. After the 2011 earthquake and tsunami, it rebuilt in a way that would protect from future disasters. Mayor Emiko Okuyama shows what was remade.

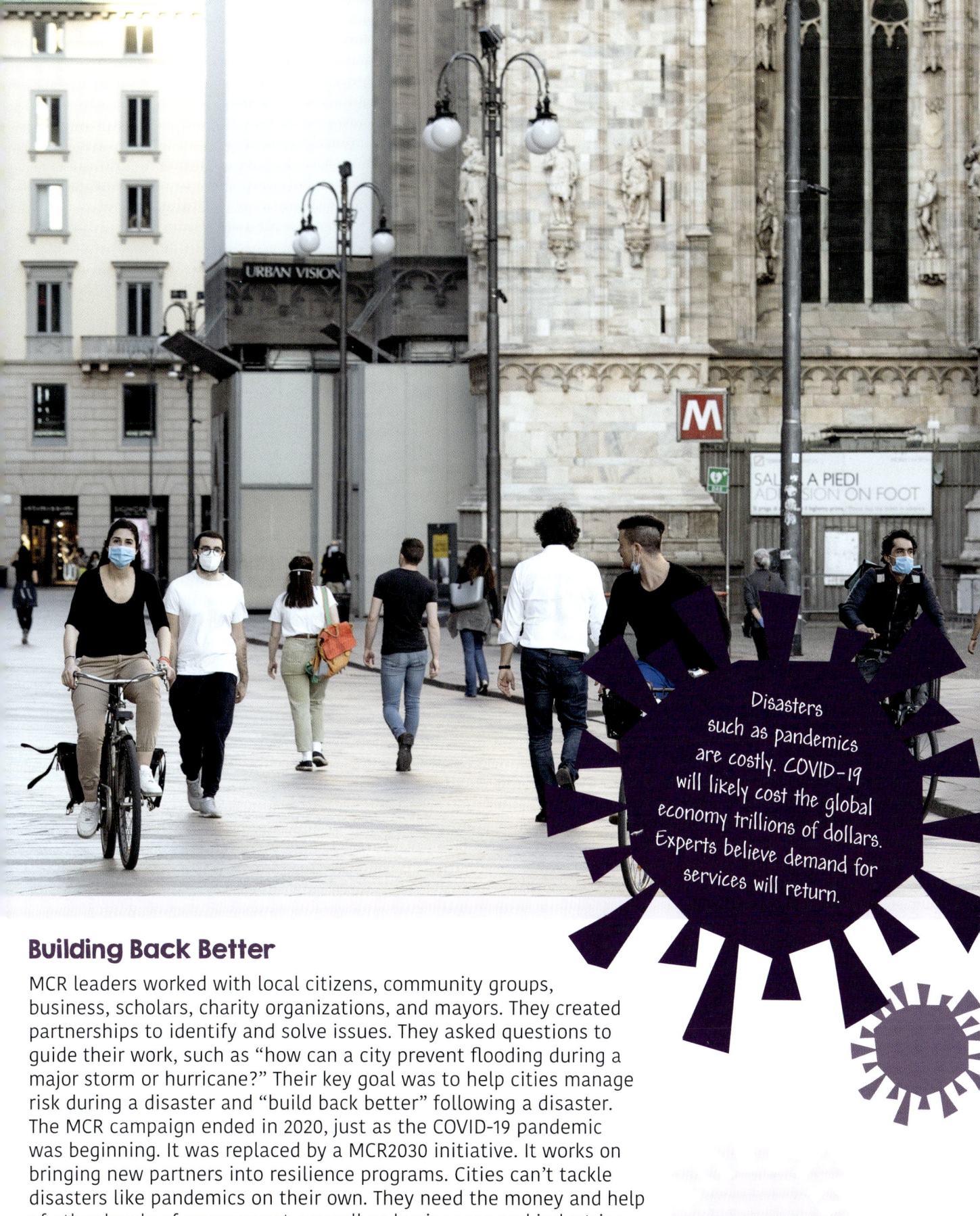

Disasters such as pandemics are costly. COVID-19 will likely cost the global economy trillions of dollars. Experts believe demand for services will return.

Building Back Better

MCR leaders worked with local citizens, community groups, business, scholars, charity organizations, and mayors. They created partnerships to identify and solve issues. They asked questions to guide their work, such as "how can a city prevent flooding during a major storm or hurricane?" Their key goal was to help cities manage risk during a disaster and "build back better" following a disaster. The MCR campaign ended in 2020, just as the COVID-19 pandemic was beginning. It was replaced by a MCR2030 initiative. It works on bringing new partners into resilience programs. Cities can't tackle disasters like pandemics on their own. They need the money and help of other levels of government, as well as businesses and industries.

Chapter 4

The 20-Minute Neighborhood

Imagine everything you need being within a 20-minute walk from home. That's the idea behind the 20-minute neighborhood. Studies have shown that most people are not willing to walk more than 20 minutes to get groceries, go to school, visit doctors, go to work, or catch a bus. Other research has suggested that at least 20 minutes of outdoor "green time" improves mental health. During COVID-19, communities around the world saw an uptick in the number of people heading outside and to parks. In one Canadian survey, 82 percent of Canadians in cities said parks became more important to their mental health during the pandemic.

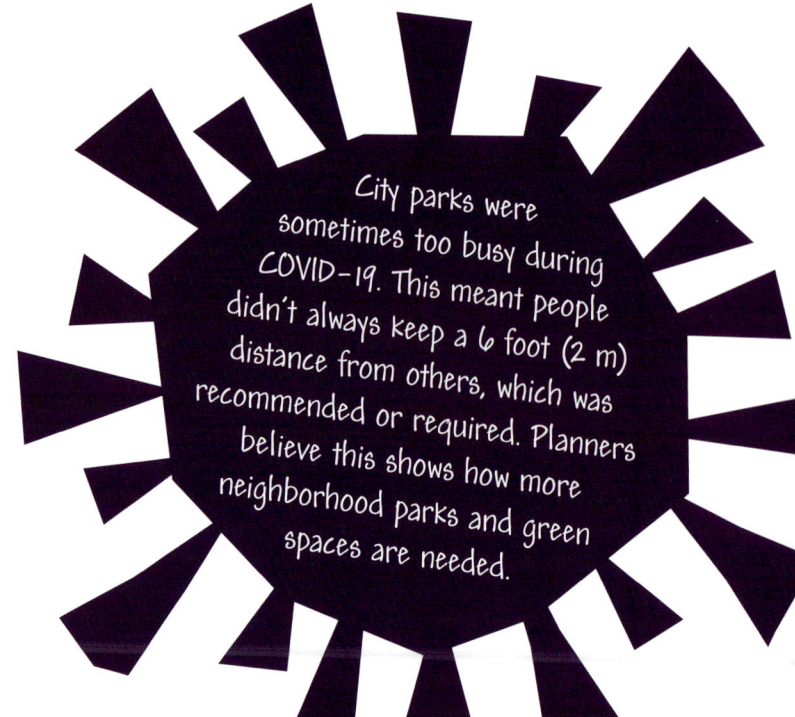

City parks were sometimes too busy during COVID-19. This meant people didn't always keep a 6 foot (2 m) distance from others, which was recommended or required. Planners believe this shows how more neighborhood parks and green spaces are needed.

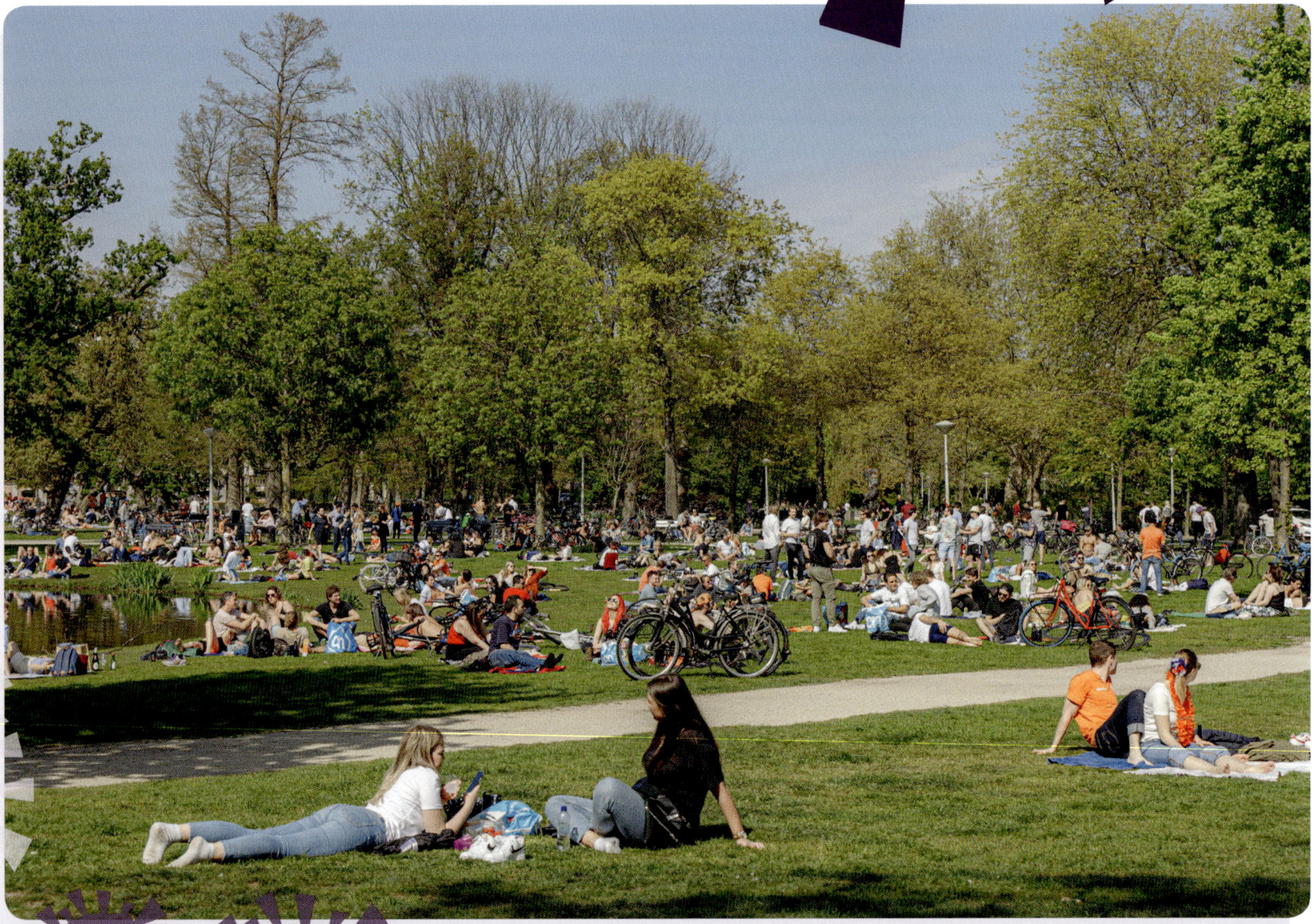

RESILIENCE STRATEGIES

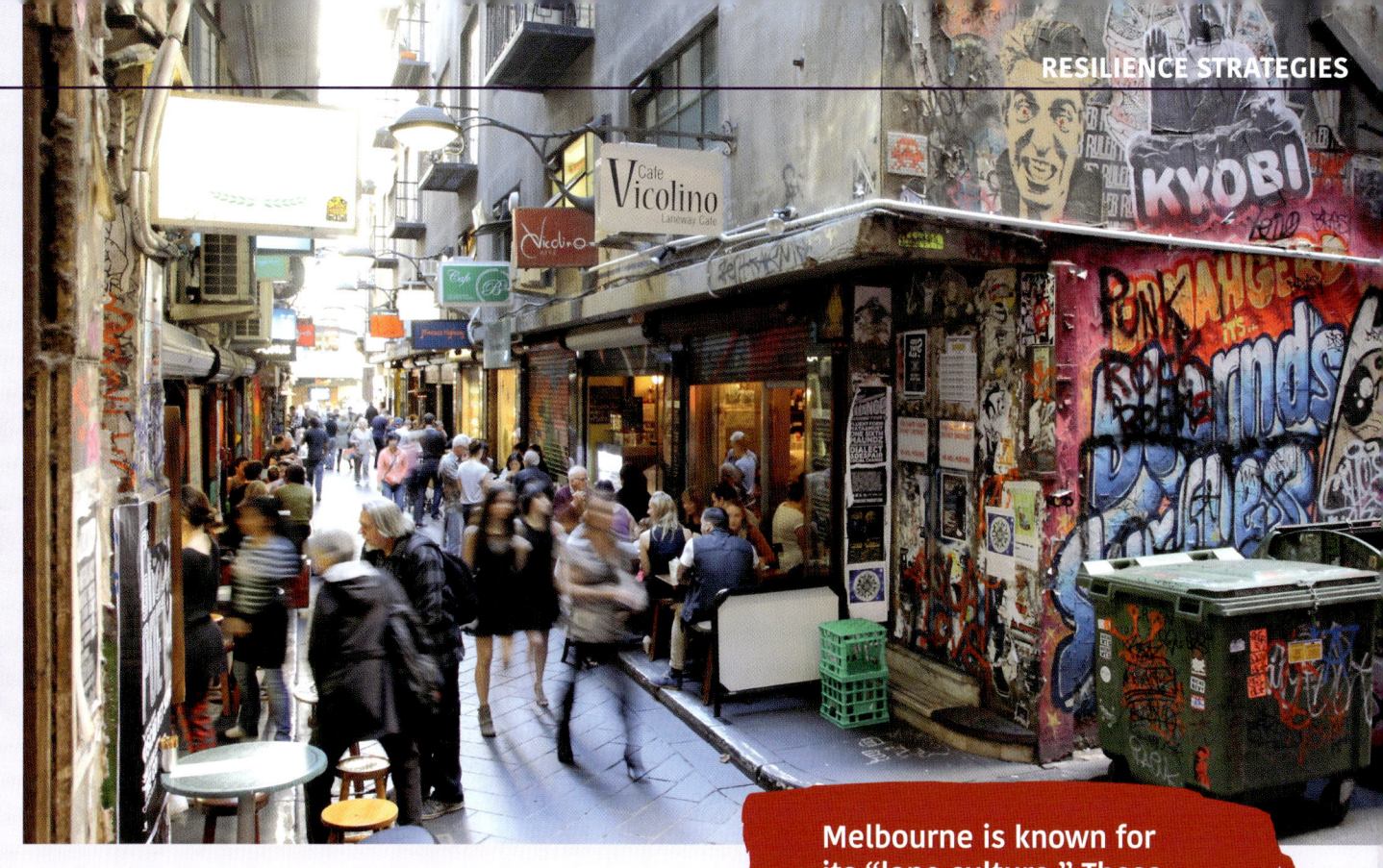

Melbourne is known for its "lane culture." These are small, walkable city streets lined with shops and restaurants. They also feature public graffiti art and attract locals and tourists.

Access Is Key

The city of Melbourne, Australia is a pioneer of the 20-minute neighborhood concept. Since 2017, city planners there have worked to build communities with schools, shops, parks, and work within 20 minutes of neighborhoods. During COVID-19, Melbourne had several strict lockdowns. One lasted 111 days. Residents were not allowed to leave their homes except for essential reasons. They also had to stay within 3.1 miles (5 km) of their homes for shopping. They could only exercise for at first one, then two hours per day. These restrictions were made easier because many people in Melbourne already lived within 20-minutes of all the services they needed.

A key to 20-minute neighborhoods is the ability to easily walk to take public transit.

Chapter 4

Characteristics of a Resilient Community

Cities and communities have responded to a variety of disasters in the past. During **World War II**, Americans planted urban gardens to grow food when food was rationed. Cities such as Tokyo and Los Angeles have designed their modern architecture to withstand earthquakes. Many cities and communities located by lakes or oceans are preparing for rising water levels brought on by climate change. But COVID-19 has presented the most severe disruption across the world in modern times. It represents both a modern-day disaster and an opportunity to build back better.

Steps to Resilience

Planning for resilience requires three steps: prevention, protection, and preparation. Prevention involves building safe and healthy cities and communities before a crisis. Protection means having clear and easy-to-use strategies to protect citizens when an emergency happens. During COVID-19, some cities and neighborhoods had lockdowns, stay-at-home orders, or curfews to reduce the spread of infection. Preparation requires cities to make sure that health care facilities are ready for an emergency and are able to quickly respond. This could include having quarantine facilities. It could also involve setting up pop-up vaccination sites and temporary care centers, such as tents, in parking lots.

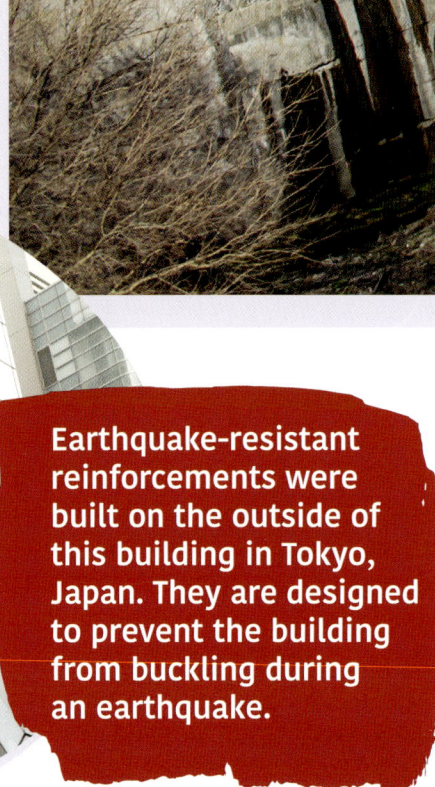

Earthquake-resistant reinforcements were built on the outside of this building in Tokyo, Japan. They are designed to prevent the building from buckling during an earthquake.

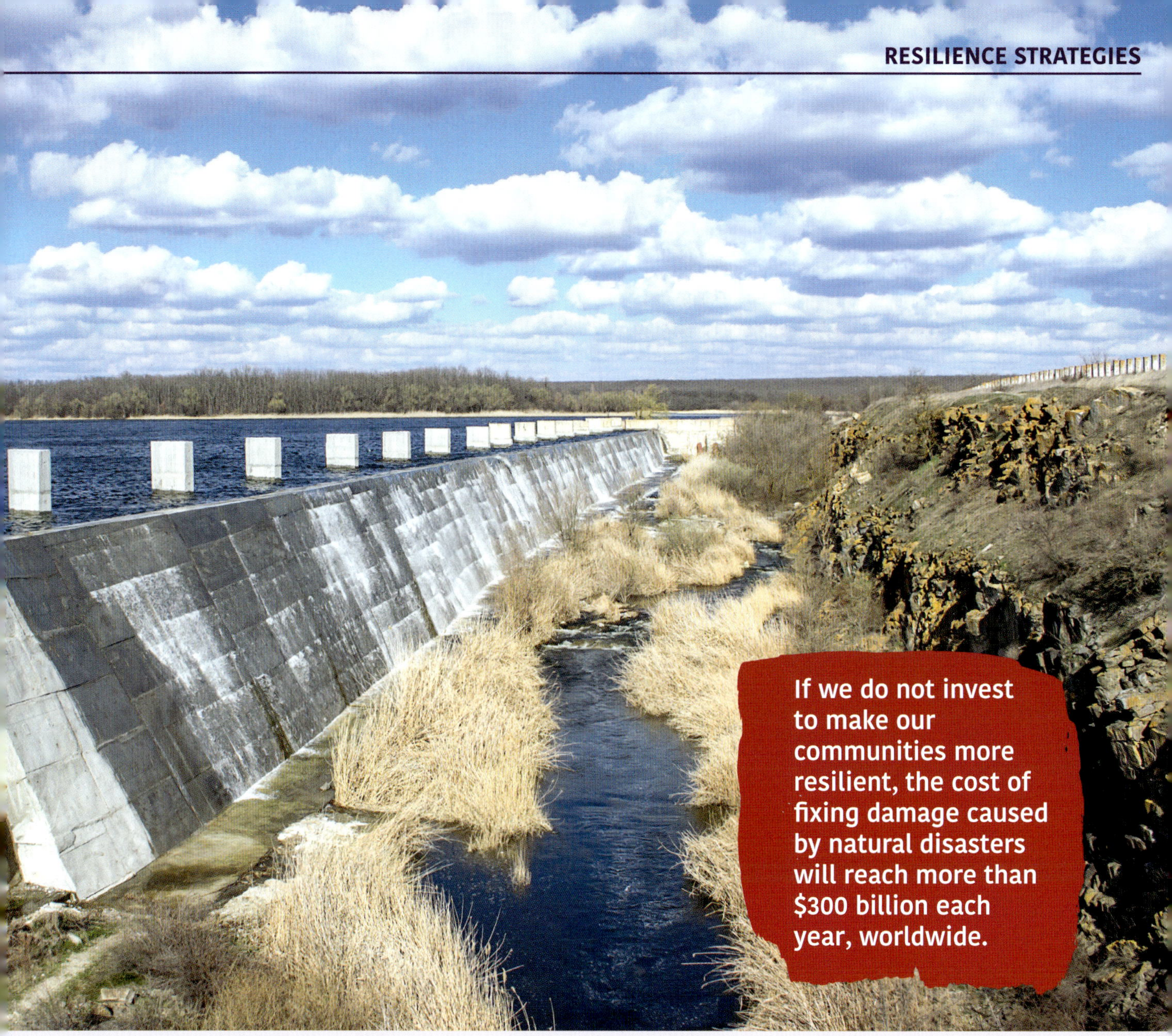

RESILIENCE STRATEGIES

> If we do not invest to make our communities more resilient, the cost of fixing damage caused by natural disasters will reach more than $300 billion each year, worldwide.

Common Characteristics

Resilient cities and communities have several common characteristics. They are reflective and resourceful. This means city officials use past experiences to help guide the way they do things. If floods always affect just one area, a city or community might strengthen flood planning in that area. Resilient communities also show strength and flexibility. They have enough supplies and resources—including emergency service people—to act during a crisis. Flexibility helps them act quickly and use a number of strategies to prevent a crisis. They have plans to use when other plans fall through. Resilient communities also ensure that the needs of all citizens are met, including the most vulnerable. If a certain part of a population routinely suffers more during a disaster, it means the city does not consider **equality** important. Many cities are actively working on changing the way things are done to build resilience.

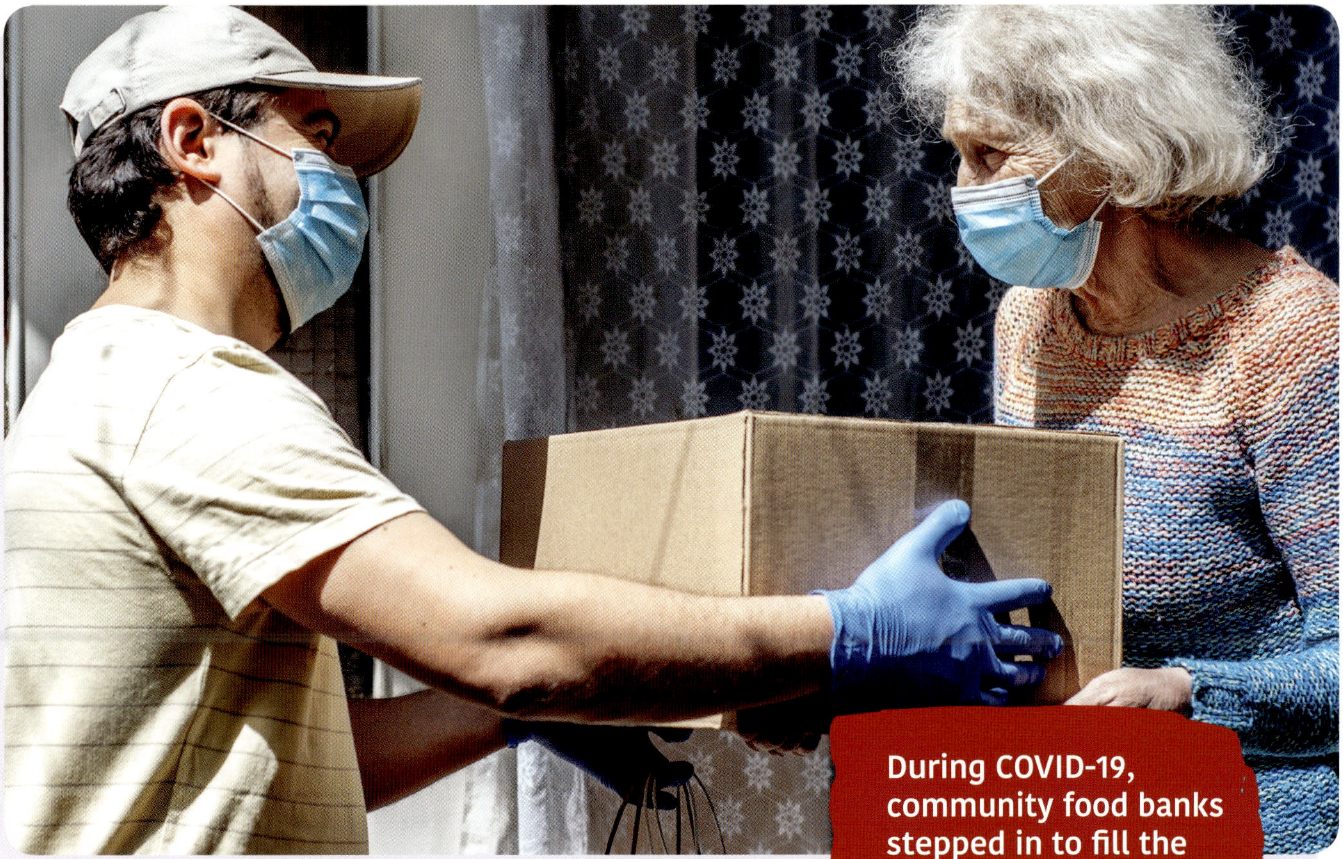

Chapter 4

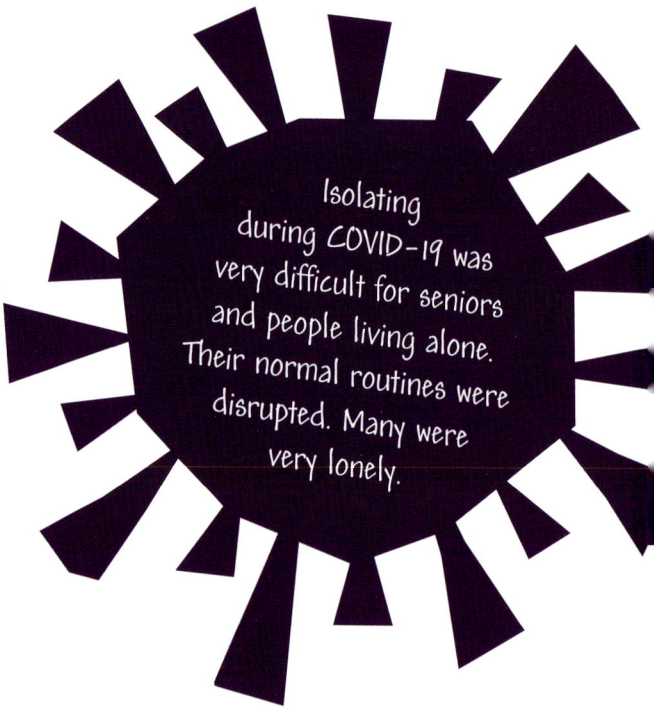

During COVID-19, community food banks stepped in to fill the gap when government supports could not.

Inequalities and Pandemics

The COVID-19 pandemic has highlighted inequalities that have existed for years in many communities. Poverty, homelessness, and **discrimination** are not new problems, but they have been made worse by this crisis. COVID-19 has shown that many people are at risk of losing their jobs or homes during a crisis. In the United States, 14 million people lost their jobs due to the pandemic in 2020. Women lost more jobs than men. Government unemployment programs helped many people. Governments also spent trillions of dollars keeping the economy steady.

Without government supports, people all over the world would be without income and homes because of COVID-19. Community-based groups have also stepped in to fill some of the gaps. They are helping support their fellow citizens in many ways. These include delivering food and medicine, volunteering at shelters, and visiting isolated individuals.

Isolating during COVID-19 was very difficult for seniors and people living alone. Their normal routines were disrupted. Many were very lonely.

RESILIENCE STRATEGIES

PANDEMIC HERO

Nicholas Scott

When his volunteer role at a senior care home was cut short due to COVID-19, Nicholas Scott was worried about how the residents would cope. He had enjoyed offering his friendship and sharing recreational activities with them, and knew they enjoyed it, too. The Grade 11 student from Ottawa, Canada, began to think of creative ways to help keep the seniors active and happy. He decided to create trivia kits and activities that could be used while he was away. He led virtual joke and storytelling sessions and called in regularly to chat with and check in on the residents. He also recorded concerts for them on his clarinet. In the spring of 2020, he performed driveway concerts for seniors in his community. One of the seniors described him as an "angel." Nicholas received a Community Builder Award for his efforts. His name was also inscribed on the Wall of Inspiration at Ottawa's City Hall.

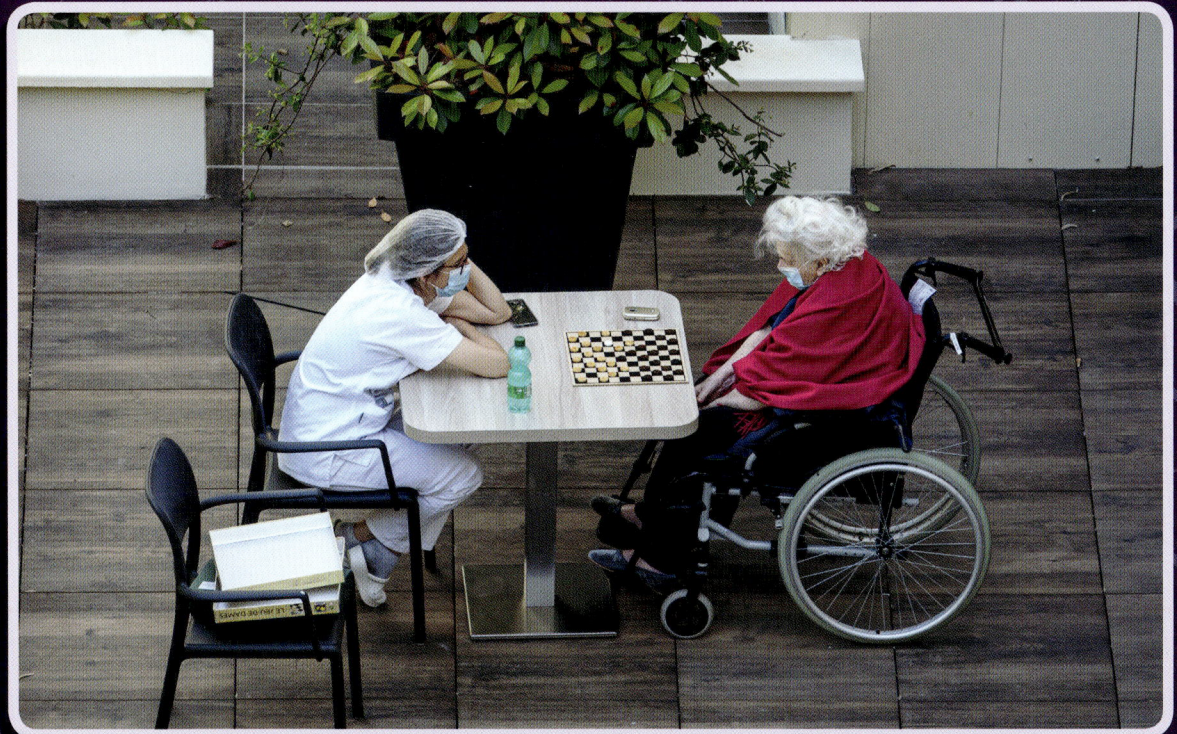

Many seniors living in long-term care homes were isolated and cut off from family and friends during the pandemic. Overworked caregivers were often their only one-on-one contact for many months.

Chapter 5

Building Resilient Communities

The strategies used to make communities resilient to pandemics will also make them safer, healthier, and fairer places to live. In many cities, where the effects of pandemics are worsened, resilience offers new help to plan for existing and future challenges. They gather and share information with others in a Resilient Cities Network.

The Resilient Cities Network is a group of cities throughout the world that have committed to making their communities less vulnerable to shocks and disasters. They share knowledge and ideas that have worked for them. Several American cities are members, including Pittsburgh, Honolulu, Houston, Nashville, New Orleans, and New York City. New York's resilience strategy is called "OneNYC 2050: Building a Strong and Fair City." It is broad and detailed. It includes plans for things such as building stronger neighborhood communities, fighting climate change, building new affordable housing, and making the city more fair. It will take some time to implement many of the changes outlined in the plan. One goal is to make the Hunt's Point Food Distribution Center in the Bronx better prepared for power outages and flooding from severe storms. It is one of the largest food-distribution centers in the world. It stores 60 percent of the city's produce and 50 percent of its meat and fish before it goes to stores. These kinds of projects are very important. They keep cities strong and **self-sustaining**.

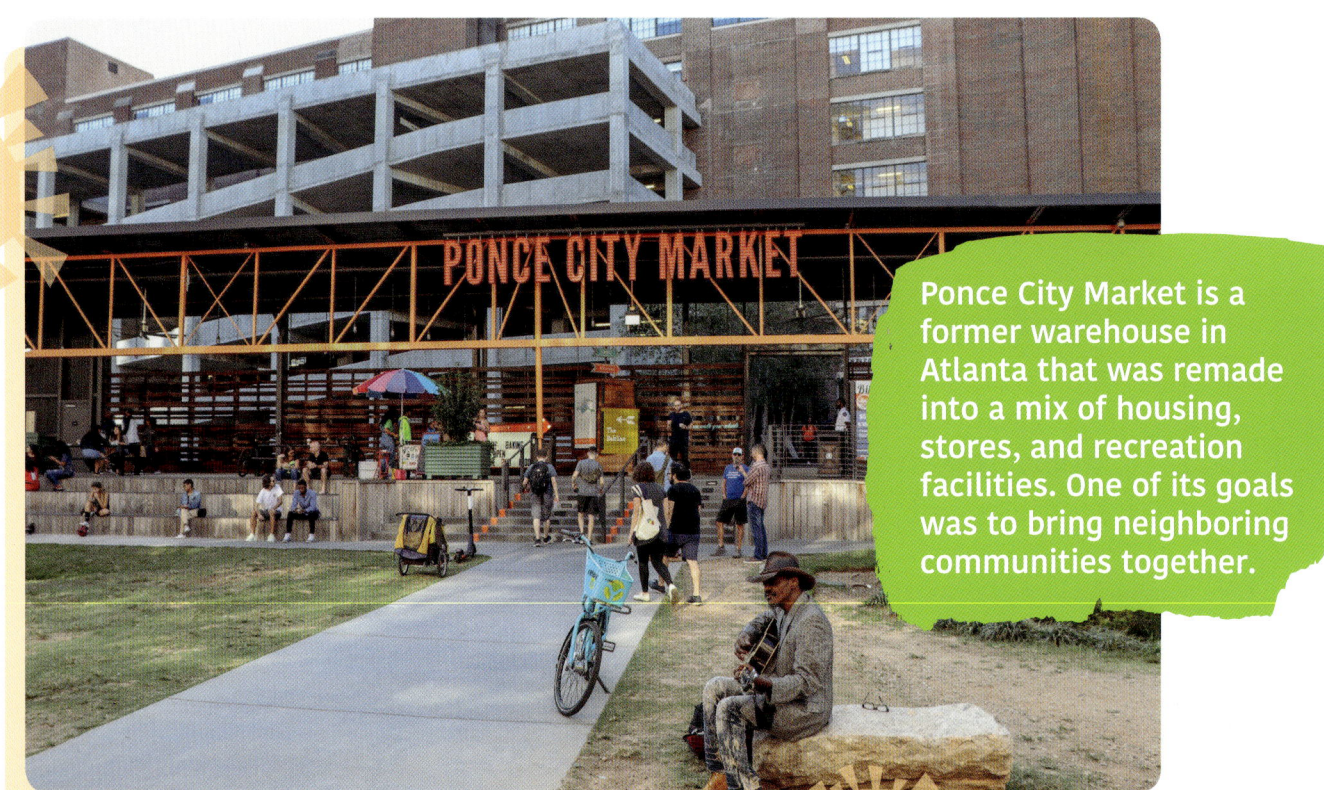

Ponce City Market is a former warehouse in Atlanta that was remade into a mix of housing, stores, and recreation facilities. One of its goals was to bring neighboring communities together.

Self-Sufficiency

Often, cities rely on supplies that have been transported hundreds or thousands of miles. These include essentials such as food and medical equipment. Closures of borders and supply routes during a crisis can cause shortages of essential supplies The COVID-19 pandemic has exposed how vulnerable cities and countries are to those shortages. Simple supplies such as toilet paper or masks were hard to get in many areas because of high demand and pressure on the supply chain. Early in the pandemic, many countries were competing for the same masks produced mostly in China.

Tech-Smart Cities

Tech-smart cities are cities that use technology to help create solutions. During the COVID-19 pandemic, smart-phone applications allowed health authorities to track the spread of infections. They used this **data** to develop quick and effective response plans. These included monitoring people to make sure they stayed in quarantine.

Programmable streets could be one future part of tech-smart cities. They could use markings that change to allow different activities throughout the day—from driving cars to pedestrian walkways or cycling lanes.

The struggle to find and purchase the masks before other countries proved how unstable some supply chains are. If a country, or community, doesn't supply some of its own needs, it must rely on the goodwill of others to get what it needs.

Chapter 5

Indoor and Outdoor Spaces

Urban parks provide city-dwellers with places to exercise, socialize, and enjoy the outdoors. During a pandemic, they can be safe spaces to socially distance with friends and family. Helping people interact with nature makes them more aware of the need to protect the natural environment. But not all city-dwellers have equal access to such spaces. Often, citizens in poorer neighborhoods and cities must travel farther to reach them.

Resilient cities include urban green spaces available to everyone. These spaces include gardens, forests, walkways, parks, and zoos.

Public Squares

City squares are often under-used spaces, crowded between skyscrapers. But they could be designed to create friendlier places for people to meet safely at outdoor cafes and on sidewalk benches. Installing public art also allows people to see and enjoy art and culture outside of crowded galleries and museums. Many cities are now embracing "pop-up" activities. These are markets, food vendors, and entertainment events that are set up in a temporary outdoor venue, such as a park or an empty lot. They provide new opportunities for people to gather safely outdoors. They can also help businesses that are shut down during a pandemic earn some money.

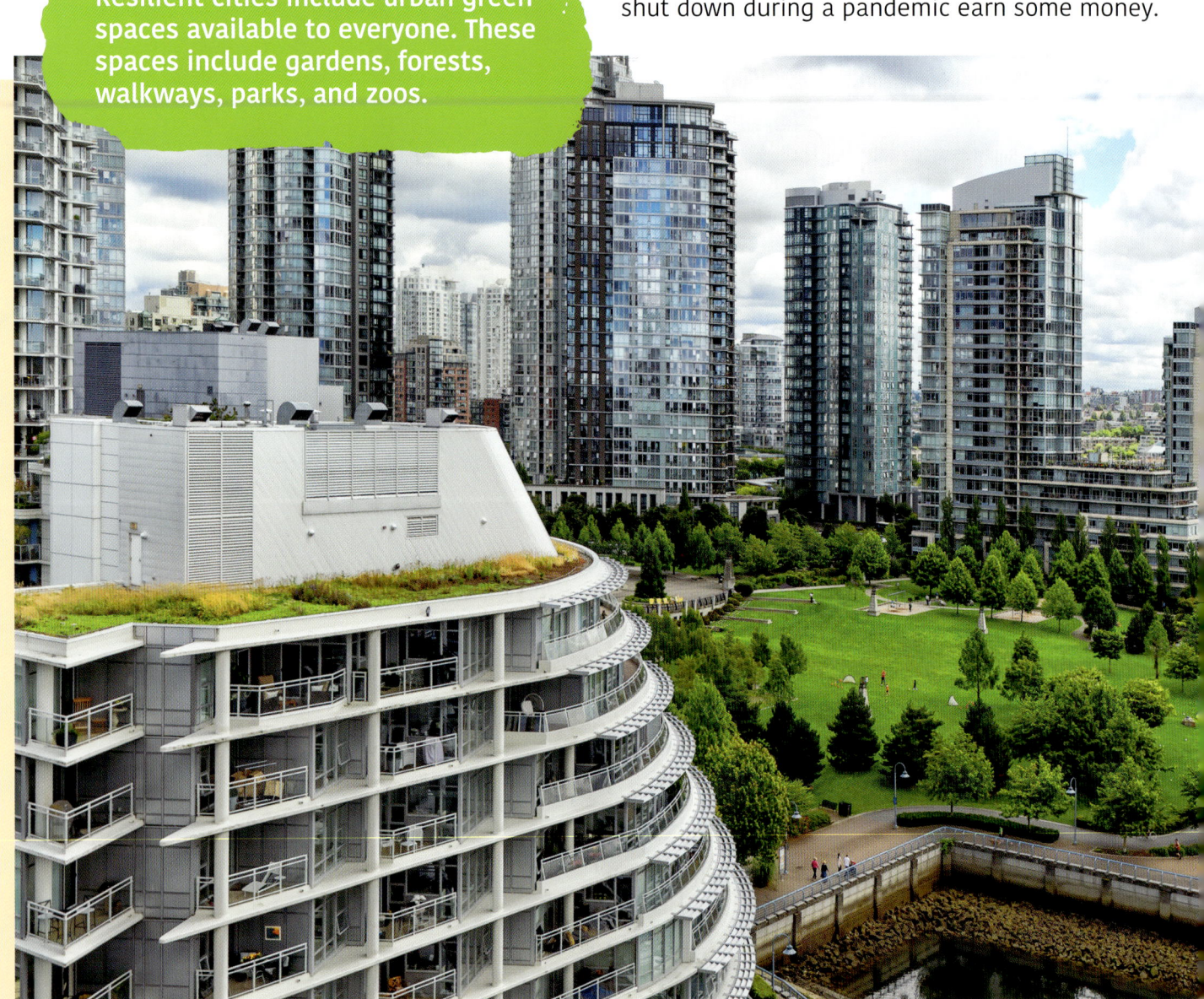

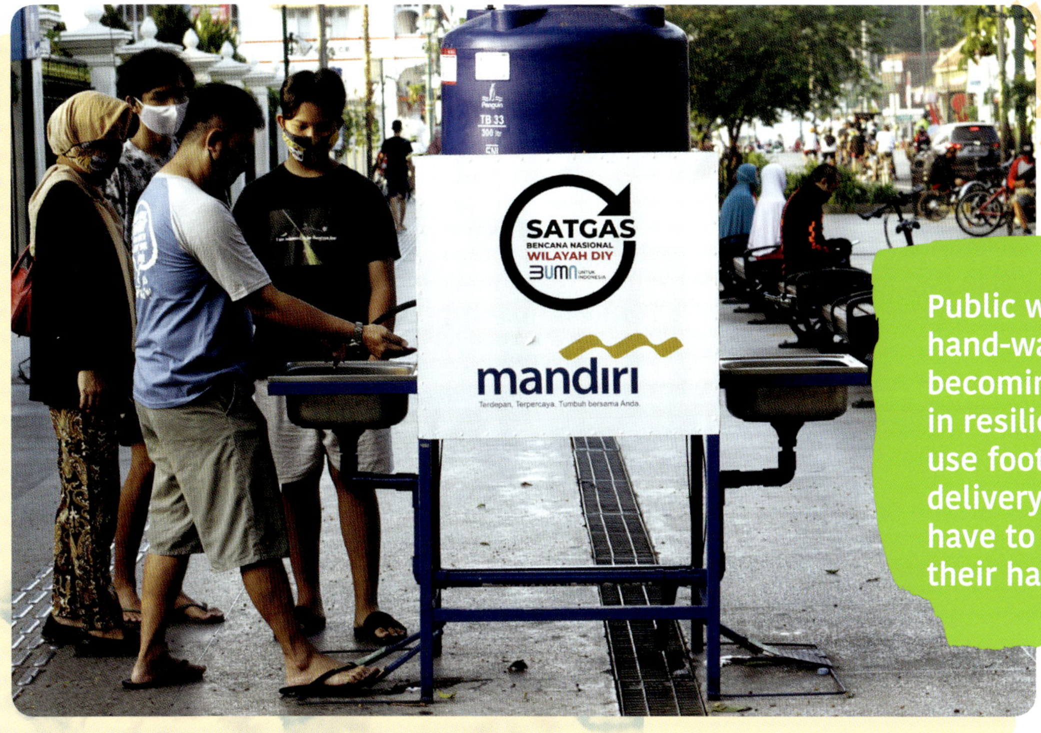

BUILDING RESILIENT COMMUNITIES

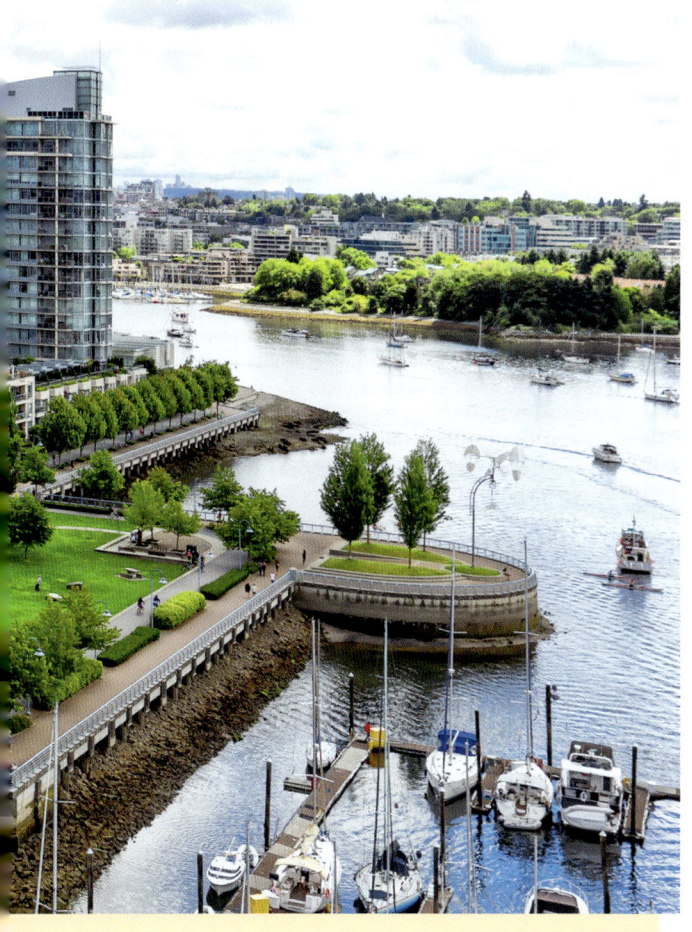

Public washrooms and hand-washing stations are becoming more available in resilient cities. Many use foot pumps for water delivery, so people don't have to touch them with their hands.

Where We Live

City buildings work best when they offer flexible spaces to live, work, and play. This is especially important during a pandemic, when many citizens are forced to socially distance or work from home. Multi-use buildings may have medical facilities, stores, housing, and flexible office spaces. They reduce the need for people to travel. They also allow people to "age in place." This means they spend their entire lives in one area, because it has everything they need.

Healthy Building Design

Building design is important. Better **ventilation** systems bring in more fresh air and help prevent the spread of disease through buildings. High-rise buildings are healthier if they have multiple elevators and staircases to reduce contact between people. Some newer buildings have stairways that are filled with light, music, and public art for people to enjoy. Rooftop and terrace gardens create beautiful spaces and allow people to grow some of their own food. The gardens also help cities reduce their **carbon footprint**.

Chapter 5

Government Actions

One thing became abundantly clear during COVID-19: countries, states, provinces, and cities need to communicate and cooperate during pandemics. Governments that provided clear, fact-based information during the COVID-19 pandemic had better outcomes. They had lower infection rates and fewer deaths. Governments that immediately shut down borders and imposed lockdowns also had fewer illnesses and deaths. Rapidly testing, tracking, and quarantining prevented the virus from spreading.

Responding Quickly

One goal of resilient communities is to respond quickly to a crisis without endangering the day-to-day needs of community members. To do this, hospitals need to have flexible spaces to help a rapid increase in patients during a crisis. Pop-up emergency spaces, such as tents or quickly refitted warehouses or stadiums, can provide additional space when needed. In Wuhan, a 1,000-bed facility was built in just ten days. In New York City, a navy hospital ship was adapted to provide care to non-COVID-19 patients. This freed up urgently needed hospital beds for COVID-19 patients. Quarantine facilities are needed to quickly isolate infected individuals to reduce the spread of disease.

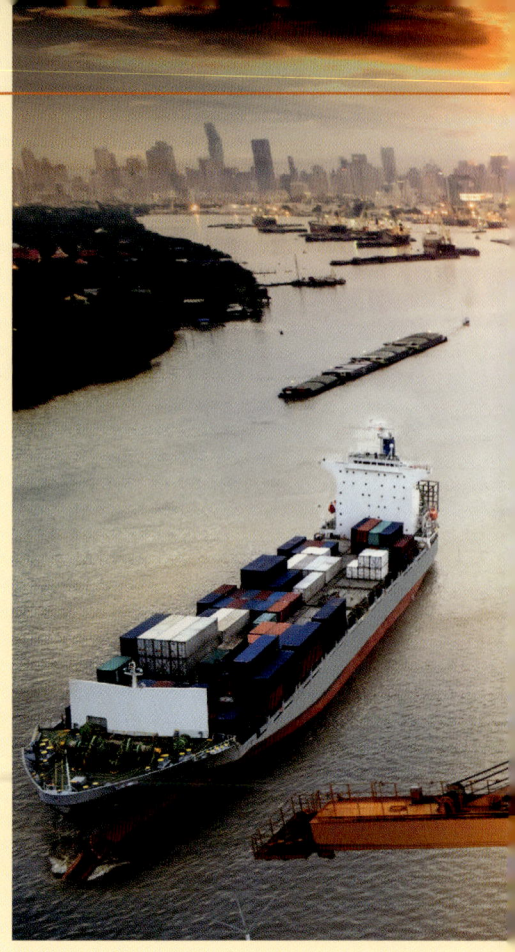

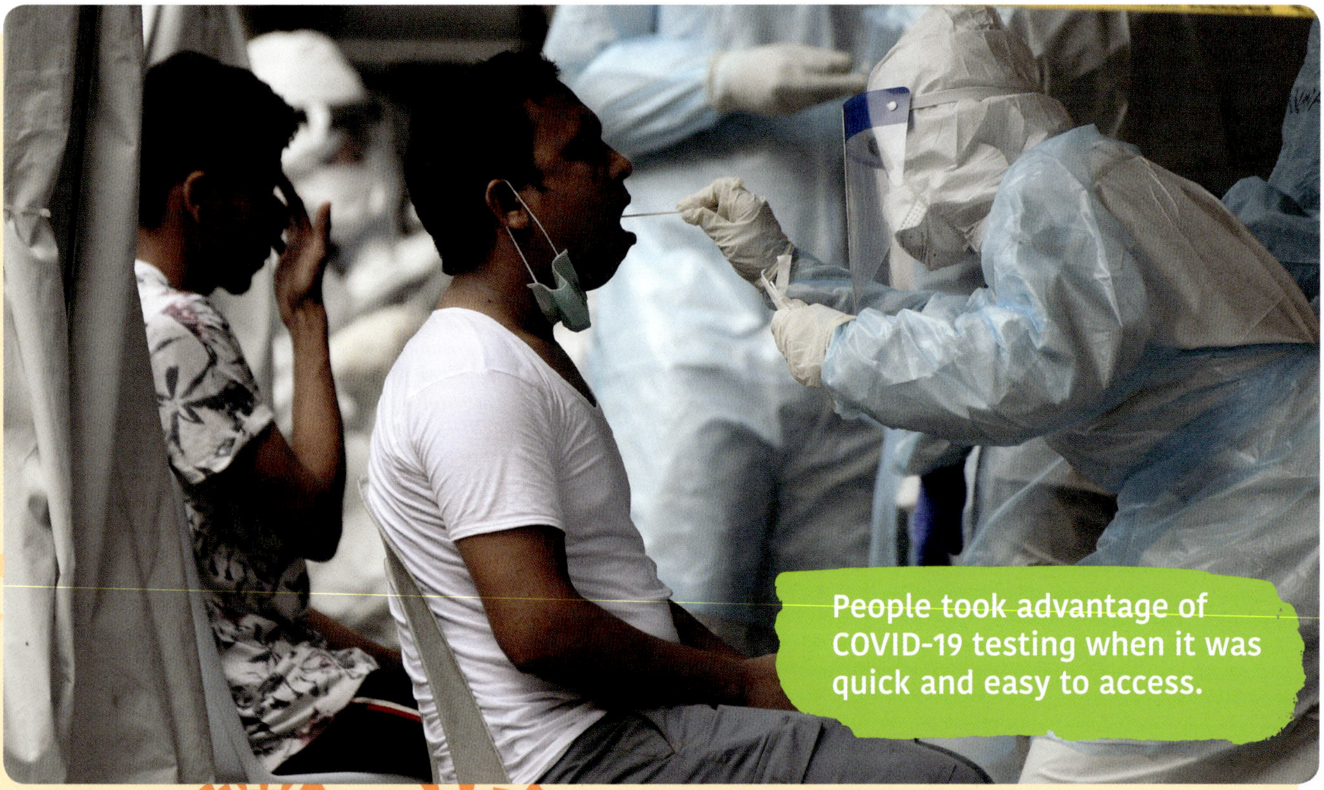

People took advantage of COVID-19 testing when it was quick and easy to access.

BUILDING RESILIENT COMMUNITIES

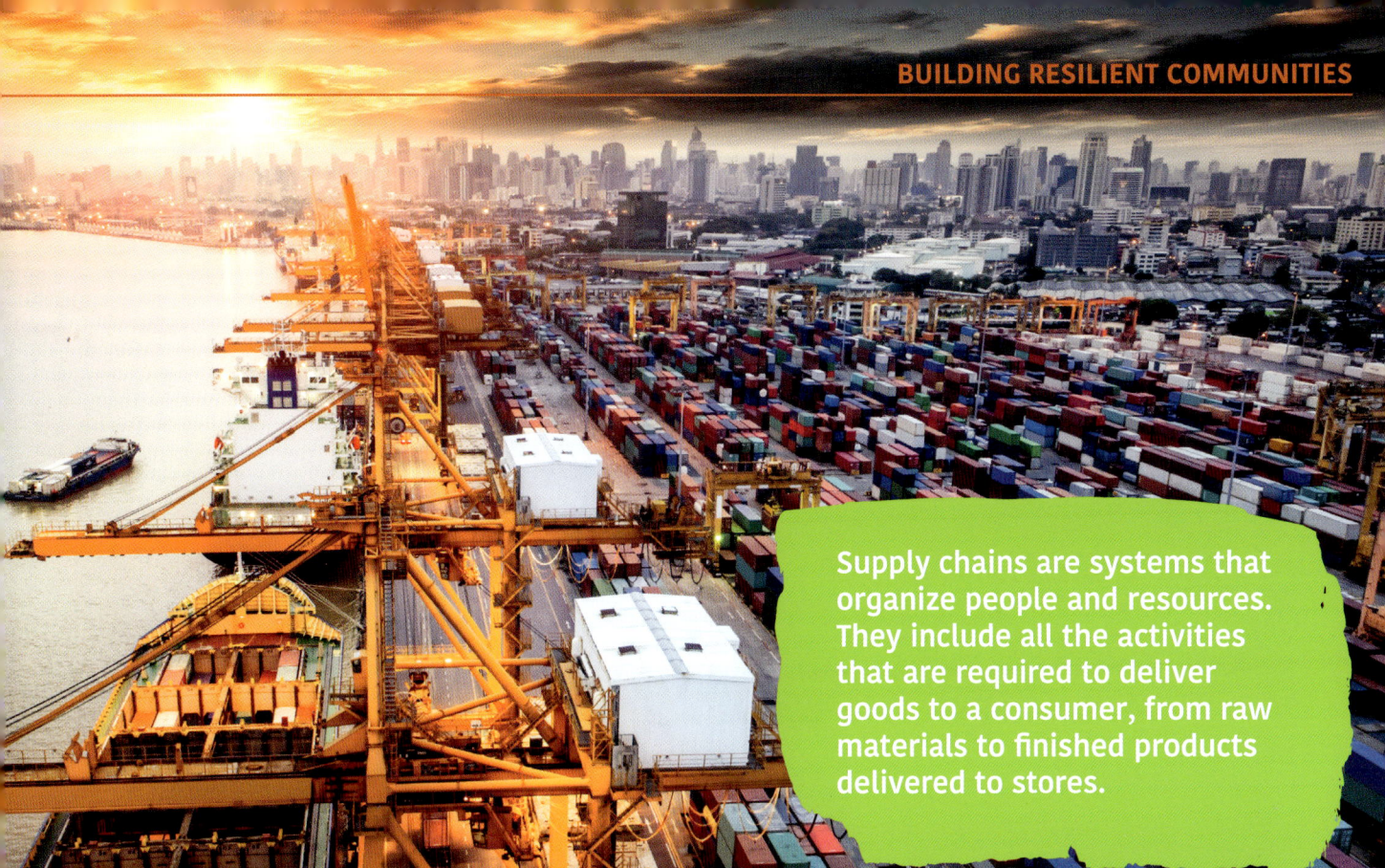

Supply chains are systems that organize people and resources. They include all the activities that are required to deliver goods to a consumer, from raw materials to finished products delivered to stores.

PANDEMIC HERO

Dr. James Mahoney

Dr. James Mahoney was known for his devotion to patient care, as well as his love of storytelling and jokes. When the COVID-19 pandemic hit, Dr. Mahoney was working at the **intensive care unit (ICU)** of the University Hospital of Brooklyn, New York. Dr. Mahoney had already been on the frontlines of the **AIDS pandemic** in the 1980s, and the September 11 terrorist attack in 2001. He was determined to provide medical care to the community that relied on the hospital, including many people in low income groups. His experience in lung disease and critical care made him especially valuable, and he refused to take even one day off. In mid-April 2020, Dr. Mahoney developed a fever and isolated at home while continuing to consult with patients. He was admitted to the hospital where he had worked almost 40 years and was later transferred to another hospital. Dr. Mahoney died of COVID-19 complications a week later, surrounded by colleagues and the medical students he helped train.

Chapter 5

Moving People

During the COVID-19 pandemic, public transit use decreased. Some people could work from home. That meant they were no longer commuting from their homes in other areas to their jobs, often in city centers. Others avoided buses and subways out of fear of contracting the virus. Although some people were driving cars into work, many were also riding bikes and walking more. In Europe and China, walking and biking increased up to 150 percent during the pandemic.

> London, England is one of many cities that have created a network of bicycle rentals to help move people around the city without cars. "Smart" traffic lights use technology to monitor traffic patterns and help cars, cyclists, and pedestrians get around more safely.

Changing Transit Landscape

COVID-19 may have kicked off new transportation trends, with cities giving more road space to cyclists and pedestrians. In Berlin, Germany, pop-up play streets were created during COVID-19 to give children a place to play outdoors. Toronto, Canada, set aside 37 miles (60 km) of "quiet streets" to create safe spaces for people to exercise on weekends. Toronto also expanded its cycling network by 15.5 miles (25 km) to ensure physical distancing during COVID-19. France introduced "Paris Respire," or "Paris Breathes" days, which eliminated cars from its city center. It also converted a highway along its famous Seine River into a riverside park. Amsterdam, Holland, turned many roadside parking spots into small community areas with plants, benches, picnic tables, and gardens.

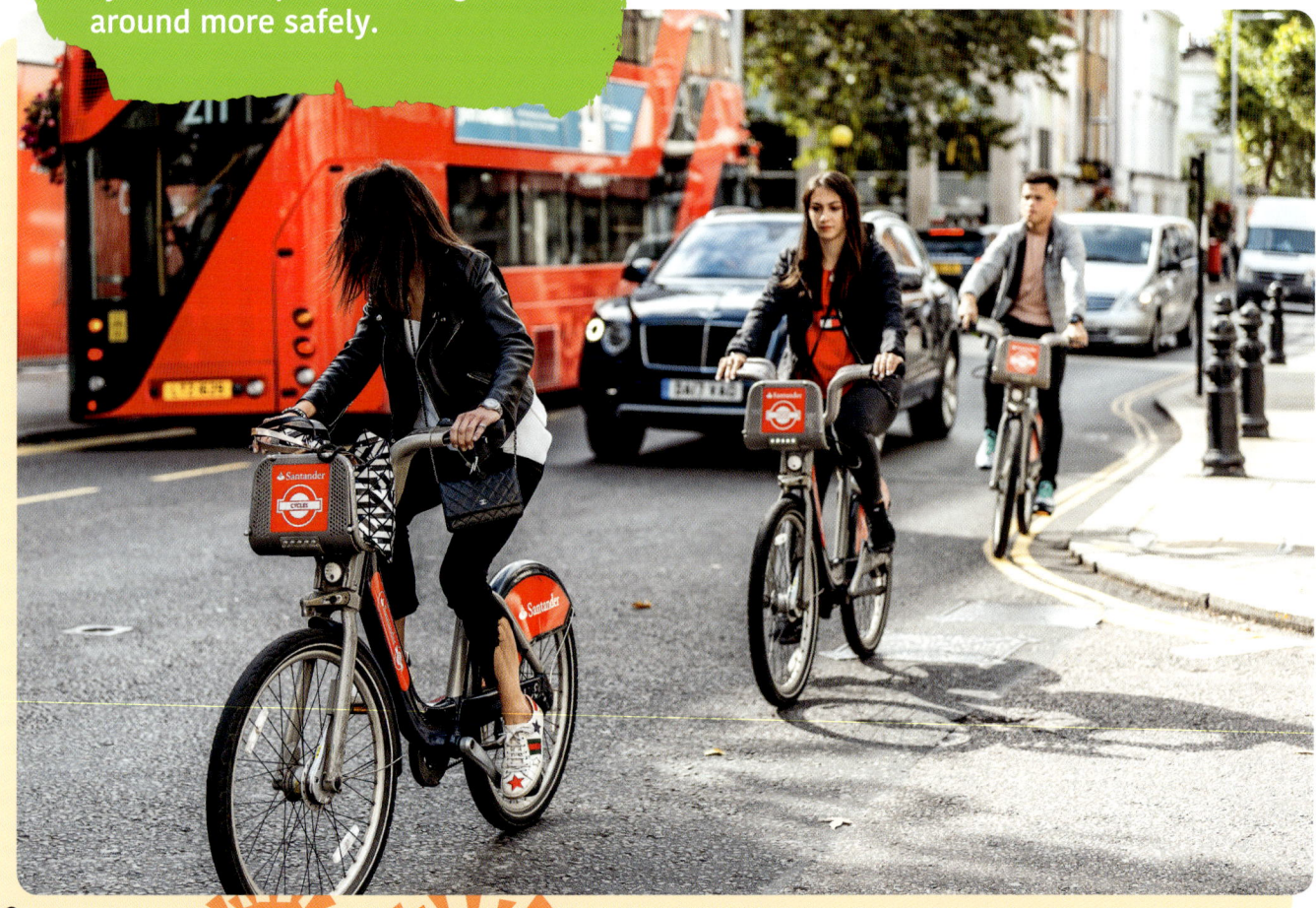

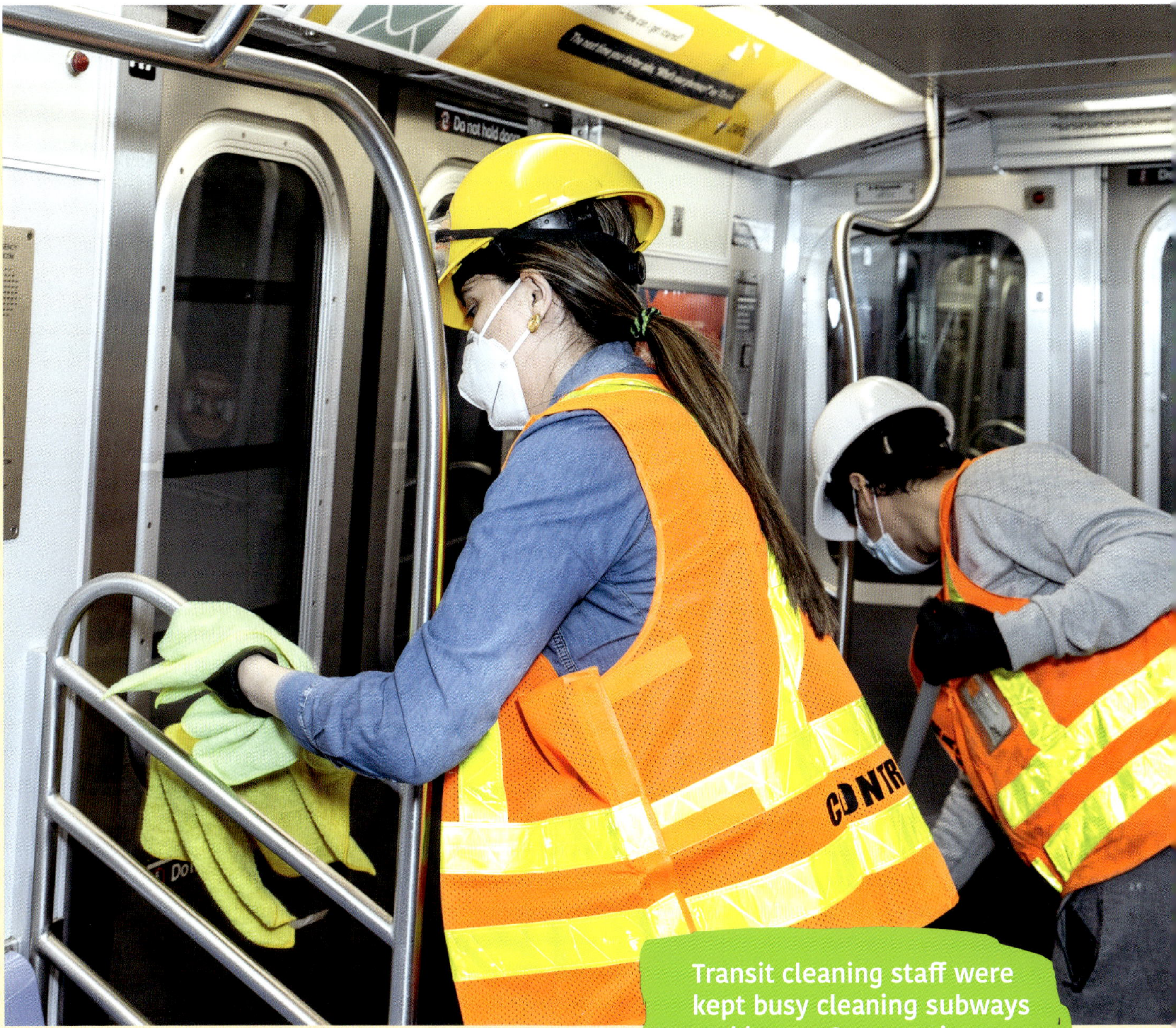

BUILDING RESILIENT COMMUNITIES

Transit cleaning staff were kept busy cleaning subways and buses. Some major cities around the world also banned eating and drinking on public transit during COVID-19. This was to ensure people wore masks to curb the spread of the virus.

Communities Need Workers

Communities depend on essential workers in order to function. Many of them rely on public transit to reach their jobs. During the pandemic, the fear of contracting COVID-19 on buses, subways, and streetcars was real. Public transit systems countered this by bumping up cleaning schedules, setting up social distance markers, and reducing hours of service. Machines that sold masks were set up in major transit stations. Some transit systems even handed out millions of free masks to encourage ridership.

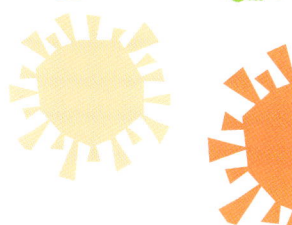

41

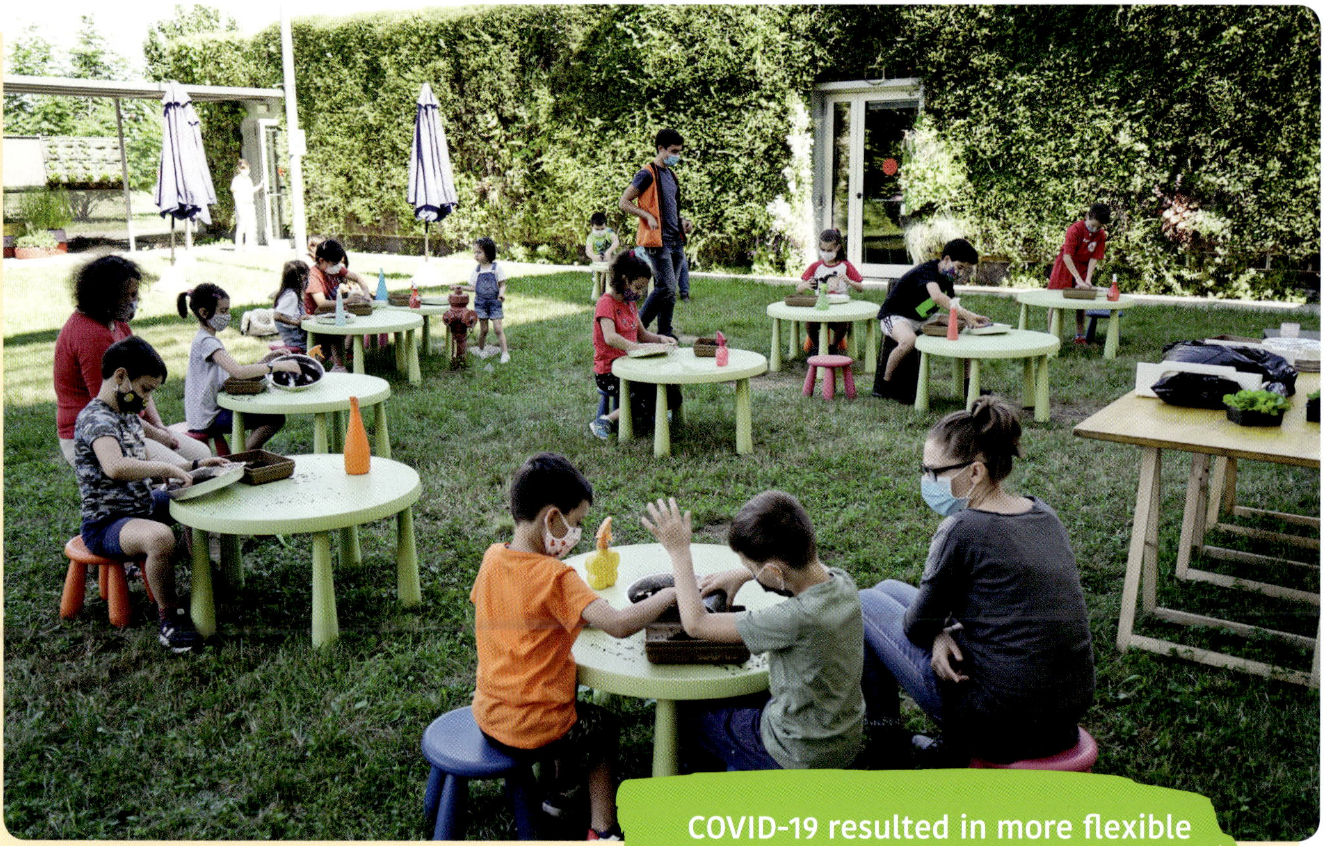

Resilient Schools

Schools were greatly affected during the COVID-19 pandemic. Some were closed altogether during lockdowns. When they were opened, many had completely changed the way they operated. The idea was to make schools safer and more resilient to the virus. In many schools, students from Grade 1 and up had to wear masks during lessons. Classes were often smaller, with desks placed apart. The COVID-19 pandemic may also change the way schools operate in future pandemics. Classrooms, schedules, and instruction times may change so they can continue with minimal disruption during any crisis. Reducing class sizes, staggering schedules, and mixing virtual and in-person learning were strategies used to protect students. These may become more common in the future.

COVID-19 resulted in more flexible learning spaces such as outdoor classrooms, gymnasiums, and field trips. These allowed students to limit close contacts while continuing their studies.

One idea for future schools is to change school designs to let in as much light and air as possible. This not only reduces the risk of disease transmission, but also helps students learn.

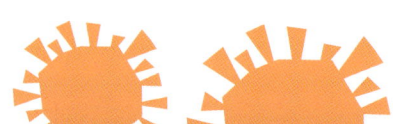

BUILDING RESILIENT COMMUNITIES

Resilient Workplaces

In most places, children's ability to attend school and their parents' ability to work are closely linked. When children are not in school, parents must stay home or arrange for child care. Strategies that enable students to remain in school with minimal disruptions play a huge role in helping parents continue to work, earn an income, and support their families. By acting quickly to control infections, governments can reduce the need for widespread lockdowns. Businesses also need pandemic plans that can be put into action quickly to support their employees. These plans could allow employees to keep working and minimize disruptions to their jobs. Work-from-home strategies have allowed many businesses to continue with full-time staff who use video conferencing to stay connected.

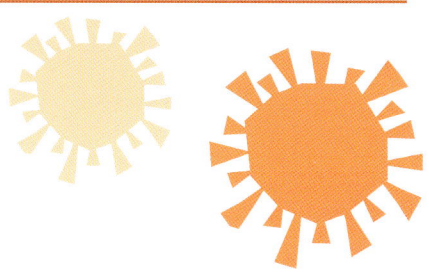

For those who continue to work in close-contact environments, safety strategies could continue in the future. These might include mask-wearing, sanitation stations, social distancing measures, and regular temperature checks.

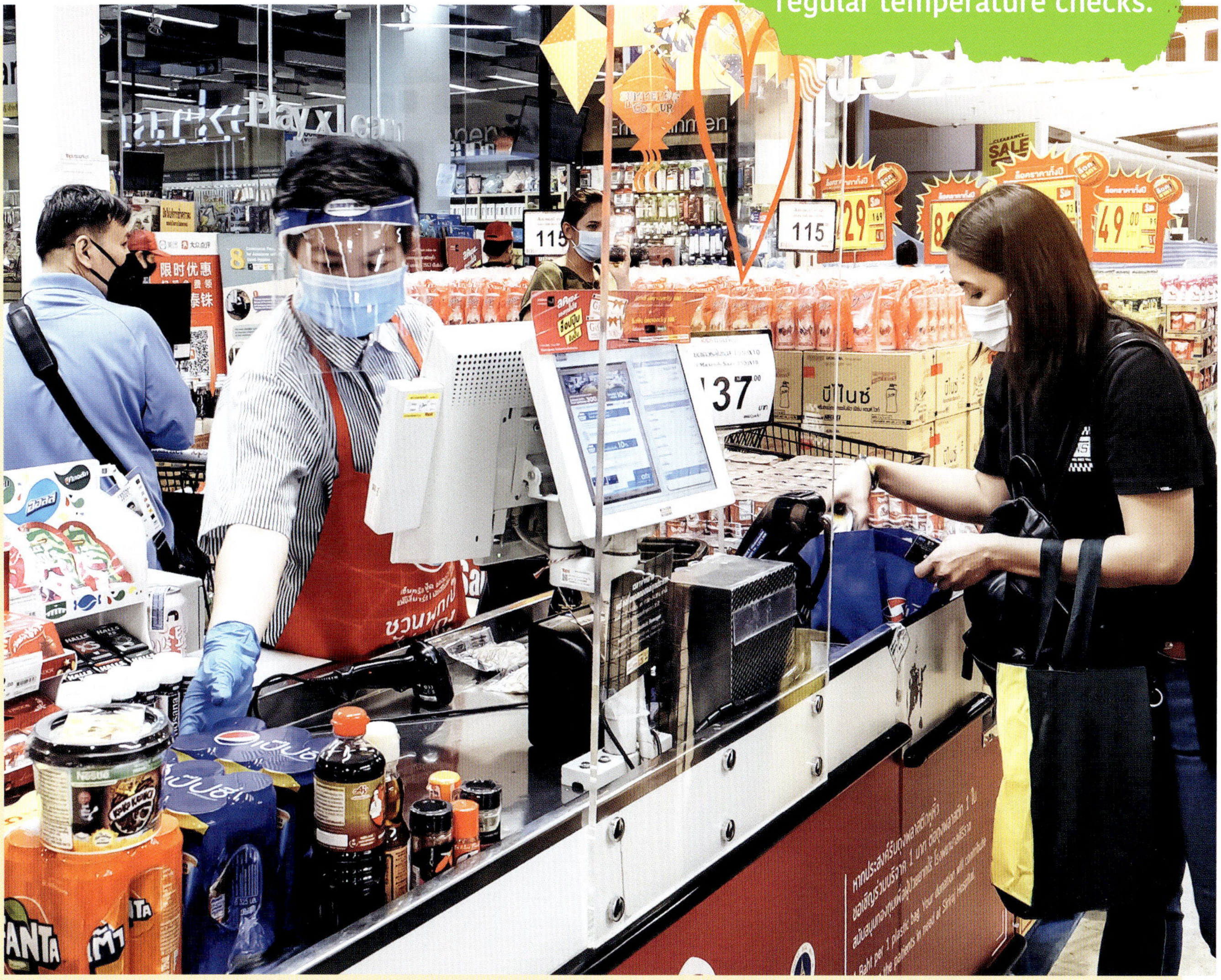

Bibliography

Intro

Graham-Harrison, Emma, and Lily Kuo. "China's coronavirus lockdown strategy: brutal but effective." The Guardian, March 19, 2020.
https://www.theguardian.com/world/2020/mar/19/chinas-coronaviruslockdown-strategy-brutal-but-effective

Chapter 1

"Ebola Virus Disease," MedBroadcast.
https://medbroadcast.com/condition/getcondition/ebola-virus-disease

Evans, Richard J. "How the coronavirus crisis echoes Europe's 19th-century cholera pandemic." NewStatesmen, April 2, 2020.
https://www.newstatesman.com/science-tech/coronavirus/2020/04/howcoronavirus-crisis-echoes-europe-s-19th-century-cholera

Glaeser, Edward L. "Cities and Pandemics Have a Long History," City Journal, Spring 2020.
https://www.city-journal.org/cities-and-pandemics-have-long-history

Kelaidis, Katherine. "What the Great Plague of Athens Can Teach Us Now." The Atlantic, March 23, 2020.
https://www.theatlantic.com/ideas/archive/2020/03/great-plague-athenshas-eerie-parallels-today/608545/

Kimmelman, Michael. "Can City Life Survive Coronavirus?" The New York Times, March 17, 2020.
https://www.nytimes.com/2020/03/17/world/europe/coronavirus-city-life.html

Riedel, Stefan. "Edward Jenner and the history of smallpox and vaccination," Baylor University Medical Center Proceedings, January 2005.
https://www.ncbi.nlm.nih.gov/pmc/articles/PMC1200696/

Chapter 2

Alter, Charlotte. "'We Won't Let Him Die in Our Ambulance.' A Day with a Paramedic Facing the Coronavirus Pandemic," Time Magazine, April 9, 2020.
https://time.com/collection/coronavirus-heroes/5815747/coronavirusparamedic-experience/

Cotterill, Joseph. "Johannesburg Covid-19 crisis: 'The storm is upon us'," Financial Times, July 14, 2020.
https://www.ft.com/content/99d6c1e3-f326-417c-8833-2dfd591d0a7b

Thompson, Derek. "What's Behind South Korea's COVID-19 Exceptionalism?" The Atlantic, May 6, 2020.
https://www.theatlantic.com/ideas/archive/2020/05/whats-south-koreassecret/611215/

Walsh, Bryan. "Covid-19: The history of pandemics." BBC News, March 25, 2020.
https://www.bbc.com/future/article/20200325-covid-19-the-history-of-pandemics

Zhu, Hengbo, Li Wei, and Ping Niu. "The novel coronavirus outbreak in Wuhan, China," Global Health and Research Policy, March 2, 2020.
https://www.ncbi.nlm.nih.gov/pmc/articles/PMC7050114/

Chapter 3

Constable, Harriet. "How do you build a city for a pandemic?" BBC Future, April 26, 2020.
https://www.bbc.com/future/article/20200424-how-do-you-build-a-city-fora-pandemic

Distasio, Jino. "How to build more resilient cities post-coronavirus," The Conversation, April 29, 2020.
https://theconversation.com/how-to-build-more-resilient-cities-postcoronavirus-136162

Mizutori, Mami, and Maimunah Mohd Sharif. "COVID-19 demonstrates urgent need for cities to prepare for pandemics," Thomson Reuters Foundation News, June 15, 2020.
https://news.trust.org/item/20200615120207-y321f

"Policy Brief: COVID-19 in an Urban World," United Nations, July 2020.
https://www.un.org/sites/un2.un.org/files/sg_policy_brief_covid_urban_world_july_2020.pdf

Puttkamer, Laura. "How Can We Make Our Cities More Resilient to Pandemics?" parCitypatory, April 25, 2020.
https://parcitypatory.org/2020/04/25/urban-resilience-pandemics/

Chapter 4

"100 Resilient Cities project," United Nations Office for Disaster Risk Reduction and the Rockefeller Foundation.
https://www.undrr.org/publication/100-resilient-cities-project

Binkovitz, Leah. "Jeff Speck, Author of 'Walkable City,' Shares His Urban Rules," Rice/Kinder Institute for Urban Research, February 27, 2019.
https://kinder.rice.edu/urbanedge/2019/02/27/jeff-speck-walkable-city-rules

"City Resilience Framework," Rockefeller Foundation, November 2015.
https://www.rockefellerfoundation.org/wp-content/uploads/100RC-City-Resilience-Framework.pdf

Clark, Greggory, Hingman Leung, Apartment613, and United Way East Ontario. "Community Builder Awards: Meet five outstanding locals who are volunteering to help others through COVID-19," Apartment613, June 13, 2020.
https://apt613.ca/community-builder-awards-meet-five-outstanding-localswho-are-volunteering-to-help-others-through-covid-19/

Garsten, Ed. "Pandemic May Accelerate Creation Of The 20-Minute City," Forbes, September 17, 2020.
https://www.forbes.com/sites/edgarsten/2020/09/17/pandemic-mayaccelerate-creation-of-the-20-minute-city/?sh=71e3238a706c

"Global Resilient Cities Network," Rockefeller Philanthropy Advisors.
https://www.rockpa.org/project/global-resilient-cities-network/

Chapter 5

"Doctor on frontline of COVID-19 battle dies in NYC." May 19, 2020. Fox10 Phoenix.
https://www.fox10phoenix.com/news/doctor-on-frontline-of-covid-19-battle-dies-in-nyc

"Facts and Figures: Urban Challenges." Urban Resilience Hub.
https://urbanresiliencehub.org/facts-and-figures/

Felter, Claire, and Lindsay Maizland. "How Countries Are Reopening Schools During the Pandemic," Council on Foreign Relations, July 27, 2020.
https://www.cfr.org/backgrounder/how-countries-are-reopening-schoolsduring-pandemic

Florida, Richard, Edward Glaeser, Maimunah Mohd Sharif, Kiran Bedi, et al. "How Life in Our Cities Will Look After the Coronavirus Pandemic," Foreign Policy, May 1, 2020.
https://foreignpolicy.com/2020/05/01/future-of-cities-urban-life-aftercoronavirus-pandemic/

Horn Phathanothai, Leo. "Towards More Equal and Resilient Cities Post-COVID-19," Global Dashboard, June 8, 2020.
https://www.globaldashboard.org/2020/06/08/towards-more-equal-andresilient-cities-post-covid-19/

Reguly, Eric. "Bikes, pedestrians and the 15-minute city: How the pandemic is propelling urban revolutions," The Globe and Mail, November 19, 2020.
https://www.theglobeandmail.com/canada/article-bikes-pedestrians-andthe-15-minute-city-how-the-pandemic-is/

Shenker, Jack. "Cities after coronavirus: how Covid-19 could radically alter urban life," The Guardian, March 26, 2020. https://www.theguardian.com/world/2020/mar/26/life-after-coronaviruspandemic-change-world

Timeline

December 10, 2019 One of the first suspected coronavirus patients falls ill in China.

December 27, 2019 Wuhan, China health officials learn that a new coronavirus is causing illnesses.

December 31, 2019 Chinese authorities alert the World Health Organization (WHO) of outbreak of pneumonia cases in Wuhan, China.

January 9, 2020 WHO announces that Chinese outbreak is caused by novel coronavirus.

January 13, 2020 First case of novel coronavirus outside China reported in Thailand.

January 21, 2020 United States confirms its first coronavirus case.

January 23, 2020 Wuhan, China is put into lockdown, but 5 million people leave the city without being screened for the illness.

February 11, 2020 WHO announces that the novel coronavirus will be named COVID-19.

March 11, 2020 WHO declares COVID-19 a pandemic and calls for global response to contain it.

April 4, 2020 More than 1 million cases are confirmed worldwide.

June 5, 2020 WHO publishes updated guidance on use of masks to control COVID-19.

September 28, 2020 The world surpasses 1 million COVID-19 deaths and 33 million cases.

October 20, 2020 A survey carried out in 19 countries indicates that 28% of respondents would hesitate to get or refuse a coronavirus vaccination.

December 8, 2020 Margaret Keenan, a UK grandmother, is the first person to be vaccinated against COVID-19 using the Pfizer vaccine approved in the UK.

January 1, 2021 The WHO approves the Pfizer vaccine for emergency use worldwide.

January 15, 2021 The world surpasses 2 million COVID-19 deaths, just four months after the first million was reached. The number of infections globally reaches 100 million on January 26.

April 9, 2021 Gibraltar (population 37,000) becomes the first country to reach 90 percent vaccination against COVID-19 for adults.

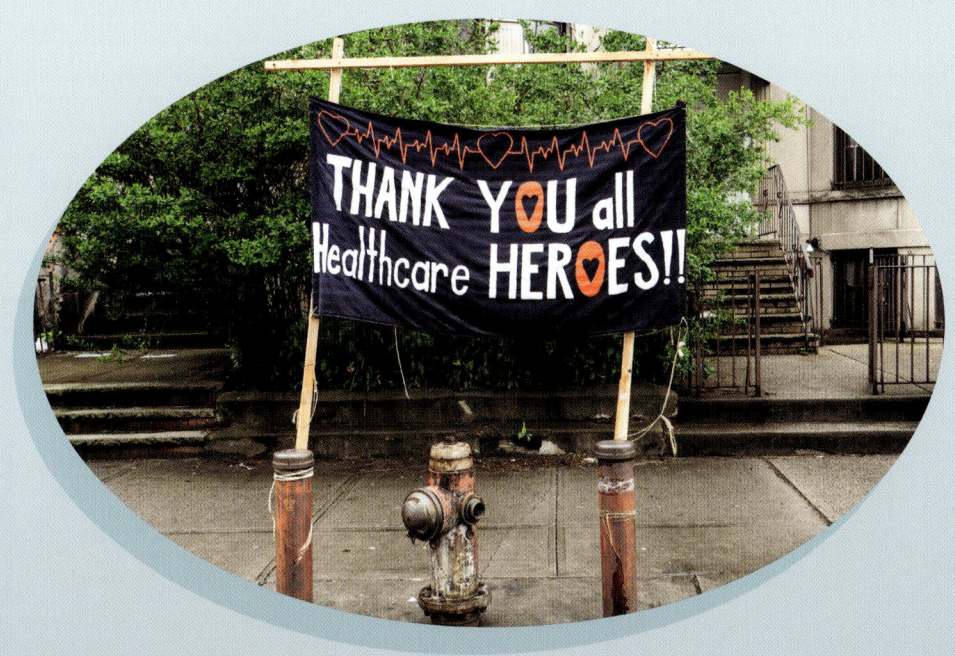

Learning More

Books

O'Brien Corasanti, Kelli, Brady Durkin, Eva Fahrenkrog, et al. *QuaranTEEN: Our New Normal: Nine Teenagers Share Their Experience of a Worldwide Pandemic*. Independently Published, August 2020.

Marcovitz, Hal. *The Covid-19 Pandemic: The World Turned Upside Down*. Referencepoint Press, 2020.

Shoals, James. *Epidemics and Pandemics*. Mason Crest Publishers, 2018.

Websites

Information on the Resilient Cities Network, its goals, and programs in various cities around the world.
www.resilientcitiesnetwork.org

Centers for Disease Control and Prevention website provides information on past pandemics and how they affected the world.
https://www.cdc.gov/flu/pandemic-resources/basics/past-pandemics.html

World Economic Forum provides an interesting visual history of pandemics and how infections are spread.
https://www.weforum.org/agenda/2020/03/a-visual-history-of-pandemics

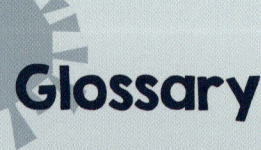

Glossary

AIDS pandemic An ongoing, worldwide epidemic of acquired immunodeficiency syndrome, a disease caused by the human immunodeficiency virus (HIV), which weakens the human immune system

carbon footprint The amount of greenhouse gases created by activities in our daily lives

cholera A serious disease that causes severe vomiting and diarrhea and can result in death

curfews A law that requires people to be indoors after a certain time at night

data Information used to study or plan something

densely populated Has a large number of people living close to one another

developed world Economically and socially advanced countries

discrimination Unfairly treating a person, or group of people differently from others

disproportionate Too large or too small in comparison with others

Glossary

economies Systems in which goods and services are made and sold in a country or region

empires Groups of nations or peoples, ruled over by one leader or government

encroaching Slowly taking control or possession of

epidemic An occurrence in which a disease spreads quickly and infects a large number of people in a country, region, or community

equality Having the same rights as others

field hospitals Temporary hospitals usually set up during war or an outbreak of a disease

first wave The first mass groups to contract the virus

inequality Not having the same rights as other people

infectious Likely to spread

intensive care unit (ICU) A special section of a hospital that treats extremely ill people

lockdown Rules put in place by the government to limit people's activities to reduce the spread of disease

nonessential Not completely necessary

nonprofit Not run for the purpose of making money

pandemic Situations in which diseases spread quickly and affect large groups of people over wide areas or across the world

public health A government service that focuses on keeping the population safe and healthy

quarantine The practice of keeping a person away from others for a certain period of time to prevent a disease from spreading

questionnaires Written sets of questions given to people to learn more about something

ration Limit the amount of something people are allowed to have or buy

rural Relating to the countryside

sanitation The practice of keeping places free from infection and disease by removing waste

self-sustaining Not requiring any extra support to continue functioning or growing

slums Densely populated areas in which many low-income people live in substandard housing

sustainability The quality of causing little or no damage to the environment, so is able to continue for a long time

transmitted Passed between people

tuberculosis A serious disease that mainly affects the lungs

unhoused Having no shelter or place to live

vaccines Substances that are injected into people or animals to protect against disease

ventilation The process of allowing fresh air to enter and move through an indoor space

virologists People who study viruses and the diseases they cause

vulnerable Easily hurt or harmed physically, mentally, or emotionally

World Health Organization (WHO) An agency of the United Nations responsible for international public health

World War II A global war that took place between 1939 and 1945, in which more than 50 million people died

Index

20-minute neighborhoods 28–29

Africa 6, 18
Amsterdam, Holland 40
animals 11, 12, 13, 14
Asia 4–5, 6, 12, 14, 40
Athens, Greece 6

Badgley, Alanna 17
Berkowitz, Michael 25
bicycles 40
Black Death/bubonic plague 6, 7, 8
businesses 4, 7, 10, 16, 20, 24, 27, 36, 43

China 4–5, 12, 14, 40, 45
cholera 7, 8
cities 8, 10–11, 16, 18, 20, 24–25, 26–31, 34–38
contact tracing/tracking 13, 18, 35, 38
contracting the virus 22, 40, 41
coronaviruses 13
cowpox 9
curfews 18, 30

deaths 6, 7, 8, 9, 12, 13, 17, 18, 19, 38, 39
disabled people 22, 23
disaster/crisis planning 24, 25, 26–27, 30, 31, 34, 35, 38, 42

Ebola 12
economies 6, 11, 16, 18, 20, 21, 26, 32
elderly people/seniors 23, 32, 33
environment 20, 21, 36
epidemics 6, 7, 8, 14, 18
essential workers 22, 41
essentials 35
Europe 6, 7, 14, 40

food banks 23, 32

France 40
frontline workers 16, 17, 22, 39

gathering in groups 20
Germany 7, 40
governments 4, 6, 12, 13, 15, 16, 18, 25, 27, 32, 38, 43

health care workers 16, 17, 22, 30, 33
homelessness 22, 32
hospitals 4, 16, 17, 19, 20, 38, 39

inequalities 18, 32
infectious diseases 8, 10, 14
information sharing 12, 14, 15, 34, 38
isolation 16, 18, 22, 23, 32, 33, 38, 39

Japan 26, 30
Jenner, Dr. Edward 9
job losses 16, 23, 32
Johannesburg, South Africa 18

lockdowns 4, 16, 18, 21, 22, 29, 30, 38, 42, 43
London, England 40

Mahoney, Dr. James 39
Making Cities Resilient (MCR) campaigns 26, 27
masks 8, 35, 41, 42, 43, 45
Melbourne, Australia 29
mental health 16, 23, 28
Middle East Respiratory Syndrome (MERS) 13
monitoring people 4, 18, 35

New Orleans, Louisiana 20–21, 34
New York 17, 19, 21, 34, 39
New York City 19, 20, 34, 38

parks and green spaces 28, 29, 36, 40
personal protective equipment (PPE) 18, 19
plague of Athens 6
planning 24, 26–31, 42
public health services 8, 15, 16
public transit 4, 20, 24, 25, 29, 40, 41

quarantine 4, 6, 7, 12, 30, 34, 35, 38

rationing 19
Resilient Cities Network 34
risks 11, 15, 17, 22, 23, 27, 32, 42

sanitation 8, 10, 20, 43
schools 4, 10, 16, 24, 29, 42, 43
Scott, Nicholas 33
self-sufficiency 35
Severe Acute Respiratory Syndrome (SARS) 12, 13
shortages 4, 8, 33, 35
smallpox 8, 9
social/physical distancing 20, 22, 28, 36, 37, 40, 41, 43
South Korea 13, 18
spreading of diseases 4, 6, 7, 12, 13, 14, 15, 16, 18, 19, 20, 22, 30, 35, 37, 38, 41
stay-at-home orders 4, 16, 18, 19, 30
strategies 24, 26–33
supply chains 35, 39
sustainability 21, 24

tech-smart cities 35
testing 13, 18, 19, 38
Toronto, Canada 40
transmission of diseases 10, 11, 12, 22, 23, 42
travel restrictions 4, 16, 35, 38

urban gardens 24, 30, 36, 37, 40

vaccinations 7, 9, 30
vaccines 9, 11, 45
virologists 26
vulnerable people 22, 23

water 7, 8, 10, 20, 21, 24
working from home 16, 20, 21, 22, 37, 40, 43
World Health Organization (WHO) 13, 14, 18, 38, 45
Wuhan, China 4–5, 14, 38, 45

About the Author

Linda Barghoorn has lived in cities on three continents—from North America to Europe and the Middle East. Each of these has helped shape her view of the world, the way we live in it, and how we can plan for a more sustainable future. She is a strong advocate for walkable cities and more accessible green spaces.